Ashgate Handbook of
Antineoplastic Agents

Ashgate Handbook of
Antineoplastic Agents

Edited by

G W A Milne

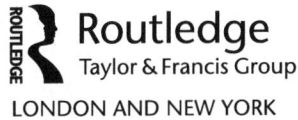

Routledge
Taylor & Francis Group

LONDON AND NEW YORK

First published 2000 by Ashgate Publishing Limited

Reissued 2018 by Routledge
2 Park Square, Milton Park, Abingdon, Oxon, OX14 4RN
711 Third Avenue, New York, NY 10017, USA

Routledge is an imprint of the Taylor & Francis Group, an informa business

Publisher's Note
The publisher has gone to great lengths to ensure the quality of this reprint but points out that some imperfections in the original copies may be apparent.

Disclaimer
The publisher has made every effort to trace copyright holders and welcomes correspondence from those they have been unable to contact.

A Library of Congress record exists under LC control number: 00104368

ISBN 13: 978-1-138-72463-1 (hbk)
ISBN 13: 978-1-138-72459-4 (pbk)
ISBN 13: 978-1-315-19237-6 (ebk)

CONTENTS

PREFACE

Chemotherapy, alongside surgery and radiation, forms the basis of modern approaches to the treatment of cancer, and has been the subject of intensive research, in academia and government for some 50 years. More recently, during the last 30 years, the pharmaceutical industry has also taken a growing interest in the development of drugs to treat cancer. As a result, several hundred chemicals have been identified as potential antineoplastic agents.

The *Ashgate Handbook of Antineoplastic Agents* contains chemical information and structures on drugs which are used in cancer treatment. This database contains 409 anticancer drugs, and 23 cytoprotectant agents which are, or have been , used in the treatment of cancer and are currently listed in the U.S. Pharmacopeia. All the antineoplastic agents contained in *Drugs: Synonyms and Properties* (also published by Ashgate Publishing Limited) are listed in this book.

Most of the records describe pure chemicals and carry the appropriate Chemical Abstracts Service (CAS) Registry Number and the associated EINECS (European Inventory of Existing Commercial Chemical Substances) number. A chemical is thus tagged with the major American and European identification numbers. In addition, all chemicals in this edition which also appear in the Twelfth Edition of the *Merck Index* have the *Merck Index* number provided. Details of the structure of a record are provided on page ix.

Proprietary Considerations

Every attempt has been made to ensure the accuracy of the information provided in the *Ashgate Handbook of Antineoplastic Agents*. However, the publishers cannot be held responsible for the accuracy of the information, and users are reminded that:

• The reporting of a name in this book cannot imply definitive legality in establishing proprietary usage. Questions concerning legal ownership of a particular name can be resolved by due legal process.

• A manufacturer in some countries may manufacture its product under names different from those cited here. Similarly, manufacture or marketing of a product may be licensed to a separate company in another country either under the same or a different name.

We trust that readers will find that this book contains a wealth of information which is difficult to obtain from any other source. It is the intention of the publishers to produce regularly updated editions and subsets of this compilation at suitable intervals in both printed and digital form. Companies wishing to submit new or updated material for inclusion in future editions should contact George W A Milne (address on page ix).

ACKNOWLEDGEMENTS

The Editor would like to acknowledge the research work performed by Dr Ellen Zeman, the skilled programming performed by Dr Ju-Yun Li which allowed for accurate formatting and typesetting of this book, and the production work which was performed by Ellen Zeman and Kay Pool.

George W A Milne
Ashgate Publishing Company
131 Main Street
Burlington VT 05401 USA
Telephone: 001-802-865-7641
Fax: 001-802-865-7847
E-mail: gmilne@ashgatechem.com

HOW TO USE THIS BOOK

The *Ashgate Handbook of Antineoplastic Agents* is divided into three Parts. A brief description of each Part is given below.

PART I

The main entries in this Part are divided into two sections:

1 Antineoplastic Agents
2 Cytoprotectant Agents

Both sections list chemical names in alphabetical order along with synonyms and other important data. Each record is identical in structure enabling the reader to select specific information efficiently. A unique record number has been assigned to every record. Indexes 1-3 in Part II allow quick cross-referencing according to the record number in Part 1 by CAS number, EINECS number, or synonym.

Record Structure

A typical record in this book is shown on the following page. The first line contains, in bold face, the record number for the record (16) and the name of the material (Alkeran Injection). The second line gives the Chemical Abstracts Service (CAS) Registry Number for the compound (148-82-3), the corresponding *Merck Index* number (5871) and the European Inventory of Existing Commercial Chemical Substances (EINECS) number

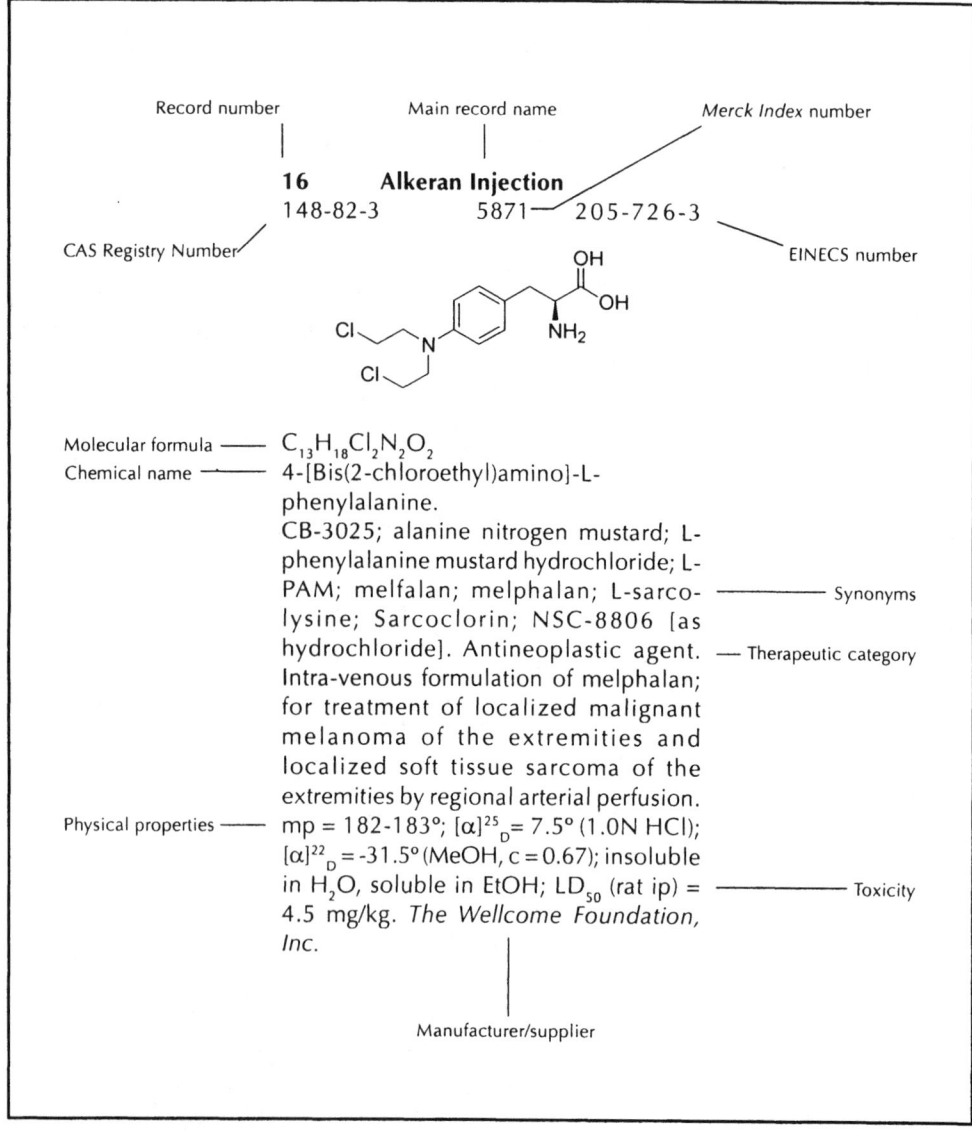

Record number   Main record name   *Merck Index* number

16   Alkeran Injection
148-82-3   5871   205-726-3

CAS Registry Number

EINECS number

Molecular formula ——— $C_{13}H_{18}Cl_2N_2O_2$
Chemical name ———— 4-[Bis(2-chloroethyl)amino]-L-
phenylalanine.
CB-3025; alanine nitrogen mustard; L-
phenylalanine mustard hydrochloride; L-
PAM; melfalan; melphalan; L-sarco- ——————— Synonyms
lysine; Sarcoclorin; NSC-8806 [as
hydrochloride]. Antineoplastic agent. — Therapeutic category
Intra-venous formulation of melphalan;
for treatment of localized malignant
melanoma of the extremities and
localized soft tissue sarcoma of the
extremities by regional arterial perfusion.
Physical properties ——— mp = 182-183°; $[\alpha]^{25}_D$= 7.5° (1.0N HCl);
$[\alpha]^{22}_D$ = -31.5°(MeOH, c = 0.67); insoluble
in H_2O, soluble in EtOH; LD_{50} (rat ip) = ——————— Toxicity
4.5 mg/kg. *The Wellcome Foundation,
Inc.*

Manufacturer/supplier

(205-726-3). These numbers always appear in the same position (left, center or right) enabling the reader to determine to which source they belong. Whenever CAS Registry Numbers are used in the text, they are always enclosed in brackets, for example [148-82-3]. The molecular formula and structure of the compound are provided and the chemical name of the compound begins on the next line. This is followed by as many as 100 synonyms, including trade names and other trivial names.

A description of the material and its known uses then follows and, when available, its physical properties are presented. These include melting point, boiling point, density or specific gravity, uv absorption, solubility and acute toxicity, usually limited to oral dosage in rodents. Finally, the companies who supply, or have supplied, the product are given.

PART II

This part contains three indexes. The purpose of each is described below:

1 CAS Registry Number Index
This index enables the reader to locate the record number and thereby find the main entry for an antineoplastic agent based on its CAS Registry Number.

2 EINECS Number Index
This index enables the reader to locate the record number and thereby find the main entry for an antineoplastic agent based on its EINECS number.

3 Name and Synonym Index
This is the master index containing all chemical and trade names found in Part I. It is the most convenient place for the reader to start if a name or synonym for a drug is known. This index enables the reader to locate the record number in Part I which relates to the main entry for that chemical.

PART III

This part contains a directory of chemical and pharmaceutical manufacturers and suppliers. Arranged alphabetically by company name, this directory provides information which will help the reader to contact the organization directly.

GLOSSARY OF UNITS

Name	Description
Mass	Unless otherwise specified, mass is expressed in a multiple of grams (g), such as micrograms (μg; $= 10^{-6}$ g), milligrams (mg; $= 10^{-3}$ g), grams (g; $= 10^{0}$ g), kilograms (kg; $= 10^{+3}$g), etc.
Volume	Volume is expressed in liters (l) or milliliters (ml) unless otherwise specified.
Temperature	When no units are cited, the temperature given is in degrees Celsius (°C).
Melting point	Melting points are cited in degrees Celsius (°C) unless otherwise specified.
Boiling point	When measured at atmospheric pressure, boiling points are cited with no pressure, e.g. bp = 167°. At other pressures, the pressure is also cited, i.e. $bp_{0.01} = 167°$.
Density	The measurement temperature is given as a superscript; thus a density of 1.123 measured at 25° will appear as $d^{25} = 1.123$. If the measurement was explicitly referenced to the density of water at 4°, the citation will carry both a superscript and a

subscript, as in $d_4^{25} = 1.123$. Specific gravities are denoted by the abbreviation 'sg'.

Optical rotation   Denoted by the letter n, refractive indexes are usually determined at a temperature which is cited as a superscript, as in $n^{25} = 1.5432$. The wavelength of the light used in the measurement is cited as a subscript, as in $n_{546}^{25} = 1.5432$. Most commonly, the sodium D line (wavelength 549 nm) is used and in such cases, the subscript is a D, as in $n_D^{25} = 1.5432$.

Refractive index   As with refractive indexes, optical rotations (α) are cited with the measurement temperature superscripted, and the measurement wavelength (often the sodium D line) subscripted, as in $[\alpha]_D^{25} = 105°$. When mutarotation can occur, the rotation given is an equilibrium value, measured after some time interval, which is cited, as in $[\alpha]_D^{25} = 105°(14\ hr)$.

UV absorption   The ultraviolet absorption maxima given by the material are cited in nanometers (nm = 10^{-9}m) and the absorptivity (E, A, ε or log ε, all of which are unitless) may also be given.

Acute toxicity   Wherever possible the units of toxicity are LD_{50}, i.e. the dose which is lethal to 50% of the test animals. In   most cases, acute toxicity is measured with the rat, orally administered, and the result is reported as LD_{50} (rat orl) = 50 mg/kg. Other species (for example, mus = mouse; rbt =   rabbit; pgn = pigeon; gpg = guinea pig; m = male; f = female) are occasionally cited as are other administration routes (sc = subcutaneous; ihl = inhalation; ip = intraperitoneal; iv = intravenous). Chronic toxicity data is not given.

ABBREVIATIONS AND SYMBOLS

abs config	absolute configuration
abs	absolute
Ac	acetyl (CH_3CO-)
ACE	angiotensin-converting enzyme
ACTH	adrenocorticotrophic hormone
AIDS	acquired immunodeficiency syndrome
alc	alcohol, alcoholic
amp(s)	ampule(s)
AMP	adenosine 5'-monophosphate
aq	aqueous
atm	atmosphere, atmospheric
bp	boiling point
BPH	benign prostatic hypertrophy
Bu	butyl
Bz	benzoyl (C_6H_5CO-)
c	concentration (g/100 ml), in rotations
C	Celsius (temperature scale)
cAMP	cyclic AMP
CH_3CN	acetonitrile
C_5H_5N	pyridine
C_6H_6	benzene
C_7H_8	toluene
cc	cubic centimeters (millitres)

CCK	cholecystokinin
CCl_4	carbon tetrachloride
CH_2Cl_2	methylene chloride
$CHCl_3$	chloroform
cm	centimeter
CNS	central nervous system
CoA	coenzyme A
d	dextro(rotatory)
d	density
dec	decompose, decomposition
dl-	racemic
DL-	racemic
DMA	dimethylacetamide
DMF	dimethylformamide
DMSO	dimethylsulfoxide
DNA	deoxyribonucleic acid
DOPA	dihydroxyphenylalanine
(E)-	(entgegen) opposite
e.g.	for example
ED	effective dose
EDTA	ethylenediamine tetraacetic acid
EINECS	European Inventory of Existing Commercial Chemical Substances
endo-	stereochemical descriptor
Et-	ethyl (C_2H_5-)
Et_2O	diethyl ether
EtOAc	ethyl acetate
EtOH	ethanol
exo-	stereochemical descriptor
F	Fahrenheit (temperature scale)
g	gram(s)
g/l	grams/liter
gal	gallon(s)
GI	gastrointestinal
gpg	guinea pig
H_2O	water
H_2SO_4	sulfuric acid
HCl	hydrochloric acid
HIV	human immunodeficiency virus
HMG-CoA	3-hydroxy-3-methylglutaryl coenzyme A
hmtr	hamster
hr	hour

HT	hydroxytryptamine (serotonin)
ihl	inhalation
im	intramuscular
ip	intraperitoneal
iPr-	isopropyl ($(CH_3)_2CH-$)
IR	infrared
iv	intravenous
kcal	kilocalories
l	liter, levo(rotatory)
λ (lambda)	wavelength
LC	lethal concentration
LC_{50}	median lethal concentration
LD	lethal dose
LD_{50}	median lethal dose
log	common logarithm
MAO	monoamine oxidase
max	maximum, maxima
Me-	methyl (CH_3-)
Me_2CO	acetone
MeOH	methanol
mg	milligram
min	minimum, minima, minute
MLD	minimum lethal dose
mp	melting point
μg	microgram
mμ	millimicron (nanometer)
mus	mouse
N	normal, normality
nm	nanometer (10^{-9})
NMR	nuclear magnetic resonance
NSAID	non-steroidal anti-inflammatory drug
NSC	National Service Center (of the National Cancer Institute)
NTP	normal temperature, pressure
o-	ortho
OD	optical density
orl	oral
p-	para
pgn	pigeon
pH	acid-base scale (log of reciprocal hydrogen ion concentration)
pK	log of the reciprocal of the dissociation constant
pOH	acid-base scale (log of reciprocal hydroxyl ion concentration)

ppb	parts-per-billion
ppm	parts-per-million
Pr-	propyl (C_3H_7-)
(R)	rectus (stereochemical descriptor)
rbt	rabbit
RNA	ribonucleic acid
(S)	sinister (stereochemical descriptor)
S-	symmetical
sc	subcutaneous
sec	second
sec-	secondary
SG, sg	specific gravity
spp.	species (plural)
STP	standard temperature, pressure
temp	temperature
tert-	tertiary
THF	tetrahydrofuran
U.K.	United Kingdom
USAN	United States Adopted Names
USP	United States Pharmacopeia
UV	ultraviolet
v/v	volume in volume
VIS	visible
viz.	namely
w/w	weight in weight
w/v	weight in volume
wt	weight
(Z)-	(zusammen) on the same side
>	greater than
>	less that
~	approximately
Å	Angstrom units (10^{-8} cm)

PART I

MAIN ENTRIES

Antineoplastic Agents

1   Acivicin
42228-92-2

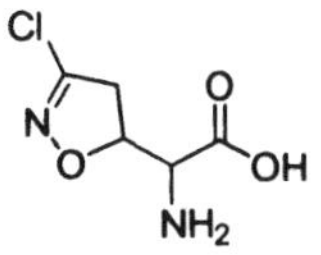

$C_5H_7ClN_2O_3$
(αS,5S)-α-Amino-3-chloro-2-
isoxazoleacetic-5-acetic acid.
AT-125; U-42126. Antineoplastic agent.
Upjohn Ltd.

2   Aclarubicin
57576-44-0   115

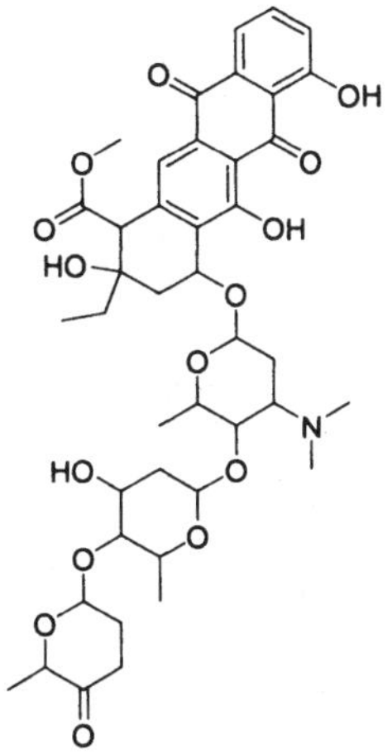

$C_{42}H_{53}NO_{15}$
2-Ethyl-1,2,3,4,6,11-hexahydro-2,5,7-
trihydroxy-6,11-dioxo-4-[[2,3,6-trideoxy-
4-O-[2,6-dideoxy-4-O[(2R-trans)-
tetrahydro-6-methyl-5-oxo-2H-pyran-2-
yl]-α-L-lyxohexopyranosyl]-3-
(dimethylamino)-α-L-
lyxohexopyranosyl]oxy]-1-naphthacene
carboxylic acid methyl ester.
Aclacinomycin   A;   NSC-208734;
antibiotic   MA   144A1;   Jaclacin.
Antineoplastic agent. mp = 151-153°
(dec); $[\alpha]_D^{24}$ = -11.5° (CH_2Cl_2 c = 1); λ_m =
229.5, 259, 289.5, 431 nm ($E_{1\,cm}^{1\%}$ 550,
326, 135, 161 MeOH), 229.5, 258.5,
290, 431 nm ($E_{1\,cm}^{1\%}$ 571, 338, 130, 161

0.1N HCl), 239, 287, 523 nm ($E_{1\,cm}^{1\%}$ 450,
113, 127 0.1N NaOH); soluble in $CHCl_3$,
EtOAc; insoluble in non-polar organic
solvents; LD_{50} mus ip) = 22.6 mg/kg,
(mus iv) = 33.7 mg/kg. *Bristol-Myers
Squibb Pharmaceutical Res. and Dev.*

3   Acodazole
79152-85-5

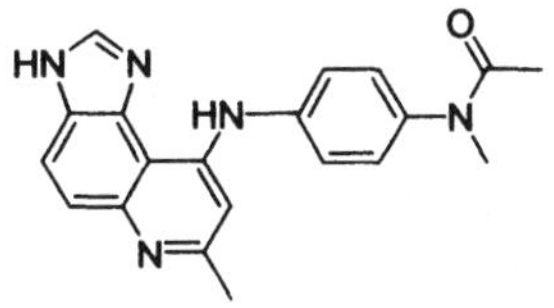

$C_{20}H_{19}N_5O$
N-Methyl-N-[4-[(7-methyl-1H-
imidazo[4,5-f]quinolin-9-
yl)amino]phenylacetamide.
Antineoplastic agent.

4   Acodazole Hydrochloride
55435-65-9

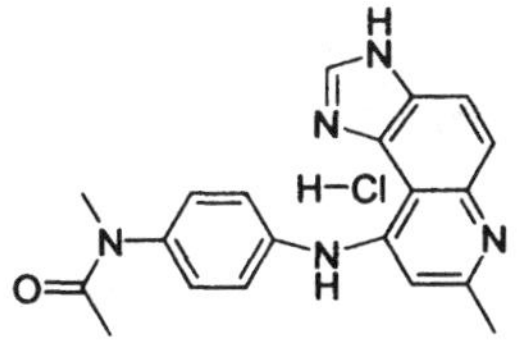

$C_{20}H_{20}ClN_5O$
N-Methyl-N-[4-[(7-methyl-1H-
imidazo[4,5-f]quinolin-9-
yl)amino]phenylacetamide
monohydrochloride.
NSC-305884. Antineoplastic agent.

5   Aconiazide
13410-86-1

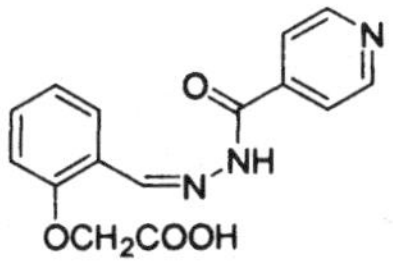

$C_{15}H_{13}N_3O_4$
Isonicotinic acid [0-(carboxymethoxy)-
benzylidene]hydrazide.
Antineoplastic agent.

6 Acronine
7008-42-6

$C_{20}H_{19}NO_3$
3,12-Dihydro-6-methoxy-3,3,12-trimethyl-[7H-pyrano[2,3-c]acridin-7-one].
Acromycine; Acronine; Acronycine; Compound 42339; NCI-C01536; NSC-403169. Antineoplastic agent.

7 Adozelesin
110314-48-2

$C_{30}H_{22}N_4O_4$
N-[2-[(4,5,8,8a-Tetrahydro-7-methyl-4-oxocyclopropa[c]pyrrolo[3,2-e]indol-2(1h)-yl)carbonyl]-1H-indol-5-yl]benzofurancarboxamide.
U-73975. Antineoplastic agent. *Upjohn Ltd.*

8 Adriamycin
25316-40-9   3495   246-818-3

$C_{27}H_{29}NO_{11}$.HCl
(8S-cis)-10-[(3-Amino-2,3,6-trideoxy-α-L-lyxo-hexopyranosyl)oxy]-7,8,9,10-tetrahydro-6,8,11-trihydroxy-8-(hydroxyacetyl)-1-methoxy-5,12-naphthacenedione hydrochloride.
Adriacin; adriablastina; Doxorubicin hydrochloride; Adrib; DOX HC; hydroxydaunorubicin hydrochloride; DOXIL; 14-hydroxydaunomycin hydrochloride; NSC-123127. Antineoplastic agent. A freeze-dried powder containing lactose and doxorubicin hydrochloride. A prescription drug for injection as an antineoplastic agent. mp = 204-205°; $[\alpha]_D^{20}$ = 248° (c = 1 MeOH); λ_m = 233, 252, 288, 479, 529 nm; soluble in H_2O, EtOH; insoluble in non-polar organic solvents; LD_{50} (mus iv) = 21.1 mg/kg. *Farmitalia, Societa Farmaceutici.*

9 Adriablastina
23214-92-8   3495   246-818-3

$C_{27}H_{29}NO_{11}$.HCl
(8S-cis)-10-[(3-Amino-2,3,6-trideoxy-α-L-lyxo-hexopyranosyl)oxy]-7,8,9,10-tetrahydro-6,8,11-trihydroxy-8-(hydroxyacetyl)-1-methoxy-5,12-naphthacenedione hydrochloride.
Adriacin; adriablastina; Doxorubicin hydrochloride; Adrib; DOX HC; hydroxydaunorubicin hydrochloride; DOXIL; 14-hydroxydaunomycin hydrochloride; NSC-123127. Antineoplastic agent. A freeze-dried powder containing lactose and doxorubicin hydrochloride. A prescription drug for injection as an antineoplastic agent. mp = 204-205°; $[\alpha]_D^{20}$ = 248° (c = 1 MeOH); λ_m = 233, 252, 288, 479, 529 nm; soluble in H_2O, EtOH; insoluble in non-polar organic solvents; LD_{50} (mus iv) = 21.1 mg/kg. *Farmitalia, Societa Farmaceutici.*

10 Adrucil
51-21-8   4219   200-085-6

$C_4H_3FN_2O_2$
5-Fluoro-2,4(1H,3H)-pyrimidinedione.

5-fluorouracil; Efudex; fluoroplex; Ro-2-9757; 5-FU; NSC-19893. Antineoplastic agent. Injectable formulation of 5-fluorouracil, an antineoplastic agent. mp = 282-283° (dec); λ_m = 265-266 nm (ϵ 7070 0.1N HCl); insoluble in H_2O; LD_{50} (rat orl) = 230 mg/kg. *Pharmacia & Upjohn, Inc. ; Hoffmann-LaRoche Inc.; Allergan Herbert.*

11   Alanosine
5854-93-3   207

$C_3H_7N_3O_4$
(-)-(S)-2-Amino-3-(hydroxynitrosamino)-propionic acid.
Antibiotic isolated from *Streptomyces alanosinicus*. Antineoplastic agent. Dec 190°; $[\alpha]_D$ = 8° (1N HCl), -46° (0.1N NaOPH), -37.8° (H_2O); λ_m 228 nm ($E_{1\ cm}^{1\%}$ 505 0.1N HCl), 250 nm ($E_{1\ cm}^{1\%}$ 630 0.1N NaOH); slightly soluble in H_2O, insoluble in the common organic solvents; LD_{50} (mus ip) = 600 mg/kg, (mus iv) = 300 mg/kg. *Gruppo Lepetit S.p.A.*

12   Aldesleukin
110942-02-4   5020
Interleukin-2.
T-cell growth factor; TCGF; Thymocyte Stimulating Factor; IL-2. Antineoplastic, antiviral agent.

13   Alestramustine
139402-18-9

$C_{26}H_{36}Cl_2N_2O_4$
Estradiol 3-[bis(2-chloroethyl)carbamate] 17-ester with L-alanine.
Antineoplastic agent.

14   Alexan
147-94-4   2853   205-705-9

$C_9H_{13}N_3O_5$
4-Amino-1-β-D-arabinofuranosyl-2(1H)-pyrimidinone.
1-β-D-arabinofuranosylcytosine; β-cytosine arabino-side; CHX-3311; U-19920; Alexan; Arabitin; Aracytidine; Aracytine; Ara-C; Cytosar; Cytosar U; Erpalfa; Iretin; Udicil. Antineoplastic, antiviral agent. mp = 212-213°; $[\alpha]_D^{23}$ = 158° (c = 0.5, H_2O); λ_m = 281, 212.5 nm (ϵ 13171, 10230, pH 2). *Ciba-Geigy Corp.*

15   Alferon
76543-88-9   5016
Alpha interferon.
alfa interferon; IFN-α; LeIF; leukocyte interferon; lymphoblastoid interferon. Antiviral, antineoplastic agent. Alpha interferon, natural (injectable form); used for the treatment of genital warts. *Interferon Sciences, Inc.*

16   Alkeran Injection
148-82-3   5871   205-726-3

$C_{13}H_{18}Cl_2N_2O_2$
4-[Bis(2-chloroethyl)amino]-L-phenylalanine.
CB-3025; alanine nitrogen mustard; L-phenylalanine mustard hydrochloride; L-PAM; melfalan; melphalan; L-sarcolysine; Sarcoclorin; NSC-8806 [as hydrochloride]. Antineoplastic agent. Intra-venous formulation of melphalan; for treatment of localized malignant

melanoma of the extremities and localized soft tissue sarcoma of the extremities by regional arterial perfusion. mp = 182-183°; $[\alpha]_D^{25}$= 7.5° (1.0N HCl); $[\alpha]_D^{22}$= -31.5° (MeOH, c = 0.67); insoluble in H_2O, soluble in EtOH; LD_{50} (rat ip) = 4.5 mg/kg. *The Wellcome Foundation, Inc.*

17   Alkeran Tablets

148-82-3   5871   205-726-3
$C_{13}H_{18}Cl_2N_2O_2$
4-[Bis(2-chloroethyl)amino]-L-phenylalanine.
Antineoplastic agent. A proprietary formulation of melphalan; for the palliative treatment of multiple myeloma and advanced ovarian adrenocarcinoma. See Alerkan Injection. *The Wellcome Foundation Ltd.*

18   Altretamine

645-05-6   328

$C_9H_{18}N_6$
N,N,N',N',N,N-Hexamethyl-1,3,5-triazine-2,4,6-triamine.
Hexalen; HMM; ENT050852; Hexastat; NSC-13875. Antineoplastic agent. mp = 172-174°; λ_m = 226 nm (ε 49400 EtOH); LD_{50} (rat orl) = 350 mg/kg, (gpg orl)= 255 mg/kg. *U.S. Bioscience.*

19   Ambamustine

85754-59-2

$C_{29}H_{39}Cl_2FN_4O_4S$
N-[3-[m-[Bis-(2-chloroethyl)amino]-
phenyl]-N-[3-(p-fluorophenyl)-L-alanyl]-L-alanyl]-L-methionine ethyl ester.
Antineoplastic agent.

20   Ambazone

539-21-9   208-713-0

$C_8H_{11}N_7S.H_2O$
p-Benzoquinone amidinohydrazone thio-semicarbazone hydrate.
A membrane-active antitumor agent.

21   Ambomycin

1402-81-9
NSC-53397. Antineoplastic antibiotic produced by *Streptomyces ambofaciens.* *Pfizer International.*

22   Ametantrone Acetate

70711-40-9

$C_{26}H_{36}N_4O_8$
1,4-Bis[[2-[(2-hydroxyethyl)amino]ethyl]-amino]-9,10-anthracenedione diacetate.
CI-881; NSC-287513. Antineoplastic agent. *Parke-Davis.*

23   Aminopterin

54-62-6   493   200-209-9

$C_{19}H_{20}N_8O_5$
N-[p-[[(2,4-Diamino-6-pteridinyl)-methyl]amino]benzoyl]glutamic acid.
Experimental antitumor agent. Also used as a rodenticide. λ_m 261, 282, 373 nm (log ε 4.41, 4.39, 3.91 0.1N NaOH). *American Cyanamid.*

24 Aminopterin Sodium
58602-66-7   493

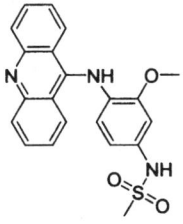

C$_{19}$H$_{18}$N$_8$Na$_2$O$_5$
Sodium N-[p-[[(2,4-diamino-6-pteri-dinyl)methyl]amino]benzoyl]glutamate.
Experimental antitumor agent. Also used as a rodenticide. *American Cyanamid.*

25 Amonafide
69408-81-7

C$_{16}$H$_{17}$N$_3$O$_2$
3-Amino-N-[2-(dimethylamino)ethyl]-naphthalimide.
Antitumor agent.

26 Amrubicin
110267-81-7

C$_{25}$H$_{25}$NO$_9$
(±)-(7S,9S)-9-Acetyl-9-amino-7-[(2-deoxy-β-D-erythropentopyranosyl)oxy]-7,8,9,10-tetrahydro-6,11-dihydroxy-5,12-naphthacenedione.
Experimental antitumor agent.

27 Amsacrine
51264-14-3   635   257-094-3

C$_{21}$H$_{19}$N$_3$O$_3$S
N-[4-(9-Acridinylamino)-3-methoxyphenyl]methanesulfonamide.
m-AMSA; CI-880; SN-11841; Amerkin; Amsidine; Amsidyl; Lamasine; NSC-249992. Antineoplastic agent. LD$_{50}$ (mus orl) = 810 mg/m^2.

28 Amsidyl
51264-14-3   635   257-094-3

C$_{21}$H$_{19}$N$_3$O$_3$S
N-[4-(9-Acridinylamino)-3-methoxyphenyl]methanesulfonamide.
amsacrine; m-AMSA; CI-880; SN-11841; Amerkin; Amsidine; Amsidyl; Lamasine; NSC-249992. Antineoplastic agent. LD$_{50}$ (mus orl) = 810 mg/m^2. *Parke-Davis.*

29 Anastrozole
120511-73-1   667

C$_{17}$H$_{19}$N$_5$
α,α,α',α'-Tetramethyl-5-(1H-1,2,4-triazol-1-ylmethyl)-1,3-benzene-diacetonitrile.

Arimidex; D-1033; ZD-1033. Antineoplastic agent. Used in breast cancer treatment. mp = 81-82°. *ICI; Zeneca Pharmaceuticals.*

30 Anaxirone
77658-97-0   278-745-8

$C_{11}H_{15}N_3O_5$
Tris(2,3-epoxypropyl)bicarbamimide.
Experimental antitumor agent.

31 Ancitabine Hydrochloride
10212-25-6   670

$C_9H_{11}N_3O_4 \cdot HCl$
(2R,3R,3aS,9aR)-2,3,3a,9a-Tetrahydro-3-hydroxy-6-imino-6H-furo[2',3';4,5]-oxazol[3,2-a]pyrimidine-2-methanol monohydrochloride.
cyclocytidine; cyclocytidine hydrochloride; cycloCMP hydrochloride; NSC-145668; OCTD hydrochloride; 2,2'-o-Cyclocytidine; 2, 2'-Anhydro-1β-D-arabinofuranosylcytosine hydrochloride. Antineoplastic agent. mp = 248-250°; $[\alpha]_D^{23}$ = -21.8° (H$_2$O, c = 2.0); λ_m = 262, 231 nm (ε 10600, 9400, pH 1-7). *Merck & Co., Inc.*

32 Ancyte
2608-24-4   7635

$C_{12}H_{22}N_2O_8S_2$
Piposulfan.
1,4-bis[3-[(methylsulfonyl)oxy]-1-oxopropyl]piperazine; NSC-47774; Ancyte; A-20968; Piposulfan. Antineoplastic agent. mp = 175-177°. *Abbott Labs.*

33 Anthramycin
4803-27-4   724

$C_{16}H_{17}N_3O_4$
3-(5,10,11,11a)-Tetrahydro-9,11-dihydroxy-8-methyl-5-oxo-1H-pyrrolo[2,1-c][1.4]benzodiazepin-2-yl-2-propenamide.
NRRL-3143. Antineoplastic agent. Isolated from *Streptomyces refuineus*. mp = 188-194°; λ_m = 235, 333 nm (ε 18200, 31800, CH$_3$CN); $[\alpha]_D^{25}$ = + 930°. *Hoffmann-LaRoche Inc.*

34 Apigenin
520-36-5   773   208-292-3

$C_{15}H_{10}O_5$
5,7-Dihydroxy-2-(4-hydroxyphenyl)-4H-1-benzopyran-4-one.

apigenine; pelargidenon 1449; Versulin; 4',5,7-Trihydroxyflavone; 5,7,4'-Trihydroxyflavone; Naringenin chalcone. A yellow dyestuff obtained by decomposing apiine, a glucoside found in parsley. A MAP kinase inhibitor. Also inhibits the proliferation of malignant tumor cells. mp = 345-350°; λ_m = 269, 340 nm (ϵ 18800, 20900 EtOH); insoluble in H_2O, soluble in EtOH.

35 Asparaginase
9015-68-3   871
L-Asparaginase aminohydrolase.
colaspase; L-asnase; E.C. 3.5.1.1.; MK-965; Crasnitin; Elspar; Kidrolase; Leunase; NSC-109229. Antineoplastic agent. $[\alpha]_D^{20}$= -31°; λ_m = 278 nm ($A_{1\,cm}^{12\%}$ 7.1 0.03M sodium phosphate at pH 7.3); soluble in H_2O, insoluble in organic solvents.

36 Asperlin
30387-51-0

$C_{10}H_{12}O_5$
5-(Acetyloxy)-5,6-dihydro-6-(3-methoxyoxiranyl)-2H-pyran-2-one.
Upjohn 224b; U-13933; NSC-93158. Antineoplastic antibiotic. Derived from *Aspergillus nidulans*. Upjohn Ltd.

37 Asulacrine
80841-47-0

$C_{24}H_{24}N_4O_4S$
9-[2-Methoxy-4-(methylsulfonylamino)-anilino]-N,5-dimethylacridine-4-carboxamide.

CI-921; NSC-343499. Potential antitumor agent.

38 Atrimustine
75219-46-4

$C_{41}H_{47}Cl_2NO_6$
Estradiol 3-benzoate 17-glycolate, 4-[p-[bis(2-chloroethyl)amino]phenyl]-butyrate.
Used as an antitumor agent.

39 Azacitidine
320-67-2   923   206-280-2

$C_8H_{12}N_4O_5$
4-Amino-1-β-D-ribofuranosyl-1,3,5-triazin-2(1H)-one.
Azacytidine; 5 AZC; 5-AC; 5-AZCR; Antibiotic U 18496; ladakamycin; U-18496; WR-183027; mylosar; Azacitidine; 5-Azacytidine; 5-AzaC; NSC-102816. Antineoplastic agent. An RNA/DNA antimetabolite. Used as an antineoplastic agent. mp = 228-230° (dec); $[\alpha]_D^{20}$ = 40° (c = 1 H_2O); λ_m = 241 nm (ϵ 8767 H_2O); LD_{50} (mus orl) = 572 mg/kg.

40   Azaserine
115-02-6   932

$C_5H_7N_3O_4$
L-Serine diazoacetate.
CI-337; CN-15757; P-165; NSC-742.
Antifungal with antineoplastic activity.
mp = 146-162° (dec); $[\alpha]_D^{27.5}$ = -0.5° (H_2O,
pH 5.18, c = 8.46); λ_m = 250.5 nm ($E_{1\ cm}^{1\%}$
1140, pH 7), 252 nm ($E_{1\ cm}^{1\%}$ 1230 0.1N
NaOH); soluble in H_2O, less soluble in
organic solvents; LD_{50} (mus orl) = 150
mg/kg, (rat orl) = 170 mg/kg. Parke-
Davis.

41   Azetepa
125-45-1

$C_8H_{14}N_5OPS$
P,P-Bis(1-aziridinyl)-N-ethyl-N-1,3,4-
thiadiazol-2-yl phoshpinic amide.
CL-25477; NSC-64826. Antineoplastic
agent.

42   Azimexon
64118-86-1   264-679-7

$C_{19}H_{14}N_4O$
1-[(1-(2-Cyano-1-aziridinyl)-1-
methylethyl]-2-aziridinecarboxamide.
Immunomodulator. Used in cancer
treatment.

43   Azotomycin
7644-67-9

$C_{17}H_{23}N_7O_8$
6-Diazo-N-(6-diazo-N-L-α-glutamyl-5-
oxo-L-norleucyl)-5-oxo-L-norleucine.
Diazomycin B; Duazomycin B; NSC-
56654.   Antineoplastic   antibiotic
produced by Streptomyces ambofaciens.
Pfizer International.

44   Batimastat
130370-60-4   1036

$C_{23}H_{31}N_4O_3S_2$
[2R-[1(S*),2R*,3S*]]-N^4-Hydroxy-N^1-[2-
(methylamino)-2-oxo-1-(phenylmethyl)-
ethyl]-2-(2-methylpropyl)-3-[(2-thienyl-
thio)methyl]butanediamide.
BB-94. Antineoplastic agent adjunct.
Antimetastatic agent. mp = 236-238°.
British Bio-Technology Ltd.

45   Benaxibine
27661-27-4

$C_{12}H_{15}NO_6$
p-(D-Xylosylamino)benzoic acid.
Potential antitumor agent.

46 Bendamustine
16506-27-7

$C_{16}H_{21}Cl_2N_3O_2$
5-[Bis(2-chloroethyl)amino]-1-methyl-2-benzimidazolebutyric acid.
Antineoplastic agent.

47 Benzodepa
1980-45-6 1118

$C_{12}H_{16}N_3O_3P$
[Bis(1-aziridinyl)phosphinyl]carbamic acid phenylmethyl ester.
AB-103; Dualar; NSC-37096. Antineoplastic agent. mp = 134-135°; insoluble in H_2O, soluble in organic solvents.

48 Besigomsin
58546-54-6

$C_{23}H_{28}O_7$
(+)-(6S,7S,Biar-R)-5,6,7,8-tetrahydro-1,2,3,13-tetramethoxy-6,7-dimethylbenzo[3,4]cycloocta[1,2-f][1,3]benzodioxol-6-ol.
A lignan component of Schizandra fruits which inhibits development of preneoplastic lesions.

49 BiCNU
154-93-8 1894 205-838-2

$C_5H_9Cl_2N_3O_2$
N,N'-Bis(2-chloroethyl)-N-nitrosourea.
Carmustine; Gliadel; BCNU; NSC-409962; Becenun; Carmubris; Nitrumon. Antineoplastic agent. mp = 30-32°; LD_{50} (mus orl) = 19-25 mg/kg, (mus ip) = 26 mg/kg, (mus sc)= 24 mg/kg, (rat orl) = 30-34 mg/kg. *Bristol-Myers Oncology*.

50 Bisantrene
78186-34-2 1284

$C_{22}H_{22}N_8$
9,10-Anthracenedicarboxaldehyde bis[(4,5-dihydro-1H-imidazol-2-yl)-hydrazone].
Antineoplastic agent.

51 Bisantrene Hydrochloride
71439-68-4 1284

$C_{22}H_{24}Cl_2N_8$
9,10-Anthracenedicarboxaldehyde bis[(4,5-dihydro-1H-imidazol-2-yl)-hydrazone] dihydrochloride.
CL-216942; ADAH; ADCA; NSC-337776; Orange Crush; Zantrëne. Antineoplastic agent. mp = 288-289° (hemihydrate); λ_m = 260, 415 nm (ϵ 72700, 16300 H_2O).

**52	Bisnafide**
144849-63-8

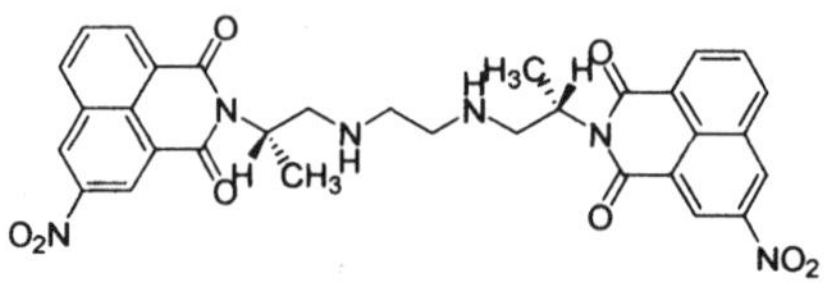

$C_{32}H_{28}N_6O_8$
[R-(R*,R*)]-2,2'-[1,2-Ethanediyl-
bis[imino(1-methyl-2,1-ethane-
diyl)]]bis[5-nitro1H-benz[d,e]iso-
quinoline-1,3(2H)-dione.
Antineoplastic agent. *DuPont Merck
Pharmaceutical Co.*

**53	Bisnafide Dimesylate**
145124-30-7

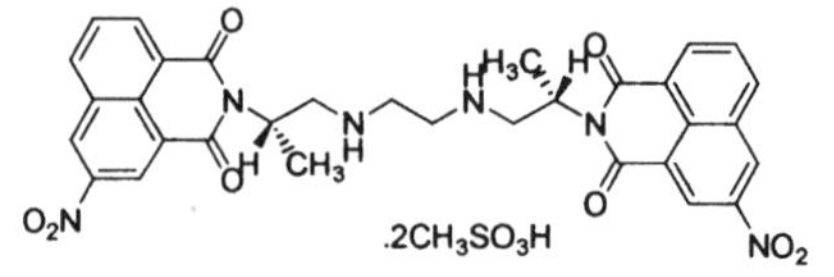

$C_{34}H_{36}N_6O_{14}S$
2,2'-[1,2-Ethanediylbis[imino(1-methyl-
2,1-ethanediyl)]]bis[5-nitro1H-
benz[d,e]isoquinoline-1,3(2H)-dione
[R-(R*,R*)] dimethanesulfonate.
VersaLuma; DMP-840. Antineoplastic
agent. *DuPont Merck Pharmaceutical Co.*

**54	Bizelesin**
129655-21-6

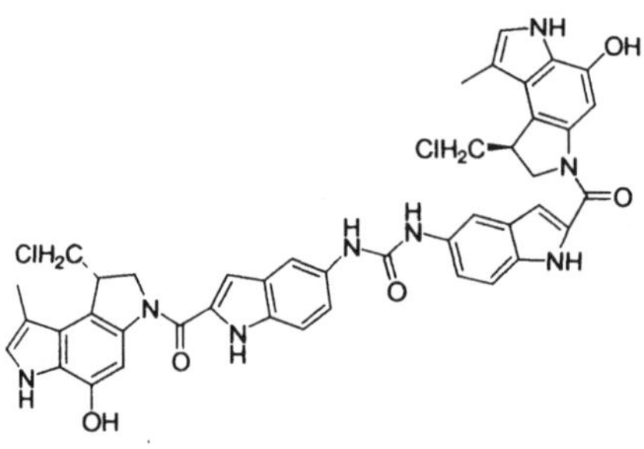

$C_{43}H_{36}Cl_2N_8O_5$
[S-(R*,R*)]-6,6'-[Carbonylbis(imino-1H-
indole-5,2-diylcarbonyl)]bis
[8-(chloromethyl)-3,6,7,8-tetrahydro-1-
methyl-benzo[1,2-b:4,3-b']dipyrrol-4-ol.

U-77779; NSC-615291. Antineoplastic
agent. *Upjohn Ltd.*

**55	Blenoxane**
9041-93-4	1351	232-925-2

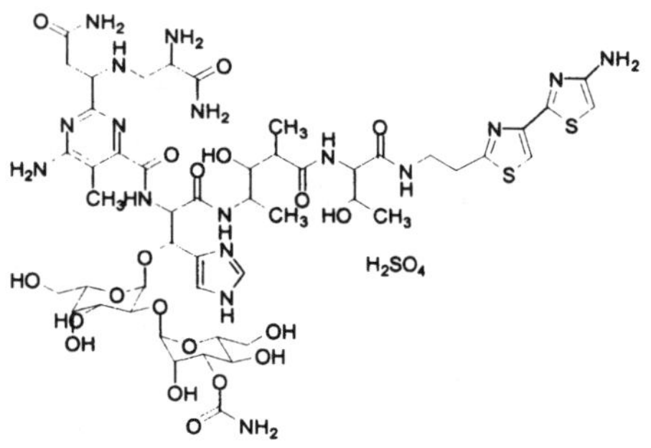

$C_{55}H_{84}N_{17}O_{21}S_3$
N^1-[3-(Dimethylsulfonio)-propyl]-
bleomycinamide.
Bleomycin sulfate. Antineoplastic agent.
Very soluble in H_2O, MeOH; slightly
soluble in EtOH; Practically insoluble in
Me_2OH, EtOAc, ether; λ_m = 244-248,
289-294 nm ($E_{1\ cm}^{1\%}$ 121-148, 102-121).
Bristol-Myers Oncology.

**56	Bleomycin**
11056-06-7	1351	232-925-2

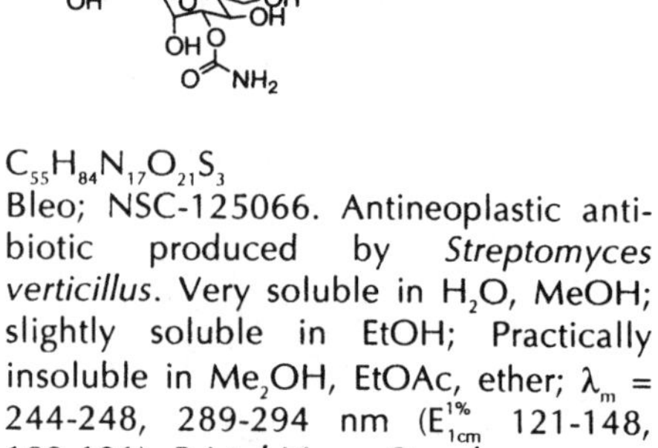

$C_{55}H_{84}N_{17}O_{21}S_3$
Bleo; NSC-125066. Antineoplastic antibiotic produced by *Streptomyces
verticillus*. Very soluble in H_2O, MeOH;
slightly soluble in EtOH; Practically
insoluble in Me_2OH, EtOAc, ether; λ_m =
244-248, 289-294 nm ($E_{1cm}^{1\%}$ 121-148,
102-121). *Bristol-Myers Oncology.*

57 Bleomycin Sulfate
9041-93-4   1351   232-925-2

$C_{55}H_{84}N_{17}O_{21}S_3$
N¹-[3-(Dimethylsulfonio)-propyl]-
bleomycinamide.
Blenoxane. Antineoplastic agent.
Antineoplastic. A mixture of
glycopeptide antibiotics isolated from a
strain of *Streptomyces verticillus* and
converted into sulfates. *Bristol-Myers
Oncology.*

58 Brequinar
96187-53-0   1394

$C_{23}H_{15}F_2NO_2$
6-Fluoro-2-(2'-fluoro-[1,1'-biphenyl]-4-
yl)-3-methyl-4-quinolinecarboxylic acid.
Biphenquinate; BPQ; DUP-785; NSC-
368390. Antineoplastic agent. mp = 315-
317°; soluble in H₂O, DMF. *E. I. Du Pont
de Nemours Inc.*

59 Brequinar Sodium
96201-88-6   1394
$C_{23}H_{14}F_2NNaO_2$
6-Fluoro-2-(2'-fluoro-[1,1'-biphenyl]-4-
yl)-3-methyl-4-quinolinecarboxylic acid
sodium salt.

Antineoplastic agent. mp > 360°; soluble
in H₂O. *E. I. Du Pont de Nemours Inc.*

60 Bromebric Acid
5711-40-0

$C_{11}H_9BrO_4$
(E)-3-p-Anisoly-3-bromoacrylic acid.
Antitumor agent.

61 Bromebric Acid Sodium Salt
21739-91-3
$C_{11}H_8BrNaO_4$
(E)-3-p-Anisoyl-3-bromoacrylic acid
sodium salt.
Cytembena. Antitumor agent.

62 Bropirimine
56741-95-8

$C_{10}H_8BrN_3O$
2-Amino-5-bromo-6-phenyl-4(3H)-
pyrimidinone.
U-54461. Antiviral, antitumor agent.
Upjohn Ltd.

63 Broxuridine
59-14-3

$C_9H_{11}BrN_2O_5$
5-Bromo-2'-deoxyuridine.
bromodeoxyuridine;   5-bromodeoxyuri-

dine; bromouracil deoxyriboside; 5-bromouracil; NSC-38297; 5-bromo-uracil-2-deoxyriboside; broxuridine; BDU; 5-BDU; BRUDR; BUDR. Antineoplastic agent.

64   Budotitane
85969-07-9

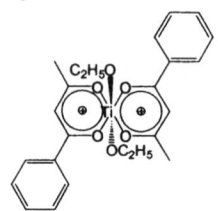

$C_{24}H_{28}O_6Ti$
Diethoxybis(1-phenyl-1,3-butane-dionato)titanium.
A titanium-containing antineoplastic.

65   Cactinomycin
8052-16-2   1642
Actinomycin C.
Sanamycin; NSC-18268. Antineoplastic.

66   Capecitabine
154361-50-9

$C_{15}H_{22}FN_3O_6$
[1-(5-Deoxy-β-D-ribofuranosyl)-5-fluoro-1,2-dihydro-2-oxo-4-pyrimidinyl]-carbamic acid pentyl ester.
Ro-09-1978/000. Antineoplastic agent.
Hoffmann-LaRoche Inc.

67   Caracemide
81424-67-1

$C_6H_{11}N_3O_4$
N-[(Methylamino)carbonyl]-N-[(methylamino)carbonyl]oxy] acetamide.
NSC-253272. Antineoplastic agent.

68   Carbetimer
82230-03-3

N-137. Antineoplastic agent. 2,5-furandione polymer with ethylene, reaction product with ammonia.

69   Carboplatin
41575-94-4   1870

$C_6H_{12}N_2O_4Pt$
cis-Diammine(1,1-cyclobutane-dicarboxylato)platinum.
Paraplatin; JM-8; NSC-241240. Antineoplastic agent. Soluble in H_2O; LD_{50} (mus ip) = 150 mg/kg, (mus iv) = 140 mg/kg; (rat iv) = 85 mg/kg. *Bristol-Myers Oncology.*

70   Carboquone
24279-91-2   1872

$C_{15}H_{19}N_3O_5$
2,5-Bis(1-aziridinyl)-3-(2-hydroxy-1-methoxyethyl)-6-methyl-p-benzoquinone carbamate ester.
carbazilquinone, Esquinone; NSC-134679. Antineoplastic agent. mp = 202° (dec); insoluble in H_2O, slightly soluble in organic solvents; LD_{50} (mus orl) = 30.8 mg/kg, (mus iv) = 6.09 mg/kg, (mus ip) = 3.84 mg/kg; (rat orl) = 28.0 mg/kg, (rat iv) = 3.88 mg/kg, (rat ip) = 3.16 mg/kg.

71 Carmofur
61422-45-5   1892

$C_{11}H_{16}FN_3O_3$
5-Fluoro-N-hexyl-3,4-dihydro-2,4-dioxo-1(2H)-pyrimidinecaroxamide.
HCFU; Mifurol; Yamaful. Antineoplastic agent. Orally active, cytostatic. mp = 110-111°; λ_m = 258 nm (ϵ 11,600 CHCl$_3$).

72 Carmustine
154-93-8   1894   205-838-2

$C_5H_9Cl_2N_3O_2$
N,N'-Bis(2-chloroethyl)-N-nitrosourea.
Bischloroethyl nitrosourea; BiCNU; BCNU; N,N'-bis(2-chloroethyl)-N-nitrosourea; N,N-Bis (2-chloroethyl)-N-nitrosourea; Bis(2-chloroethyl)nitrosourea; Carmubris; Carmustin; FDA 0345; Nitrumon; NSC-409962; NSC-409962; SK-27702; SRI-1720; 1,3-Bis(β-chloro-ethyl)-1-nitrosourea; 1,3-Bis(2-chloro-ethyl)-1-nitrosourea; 1,3-Bis(2-chloroethyl)nitrosourea. Antineoplastic agent. mp = 30-32°; soluble in H$_2$O (4 mg/ml), more soluble in organic solvents; LD$_{50}$ (rat orl) = 30-34 mg/kg.

73 Carubicin
50935-04-1   1921

$C_{26}H_{27}NO_{10}$
(8S-cis)-8-Acetyl-10-[(3-amino-2,3,6-

trideoxy-α-L-lyxo-hexopyranosyl)oxy]-7,8,9,10-tetrahydro-1,6,8,11-tetrahydroxy-5,12-naphthacenedione.
Carminomicin I; Carminomycin; Carminomycin I; Carubicin; Karminomitsin; NSC-180024. Antineoplastic agent. Anthracycline antibiotic isolated from Actinomadura carminata.

74 Carubicin Hydrochloride
52794-97-5   1921

$C_{26}H_{28}ClNO_{10}$
(8S-cis)-8-Acetyl-10-[(3-amino-2,3,6-trideoxy-α-L-lyxo-hexopyranosyl)oxy]-7,8,9,10-tetrahydro-1,6,8,11-tetrahydroxy-5,12-naphthacenedione hydrochloride.
Carminomycin hydrochloride; Carubicin hydrochloride; Karminomycin hydrochloride. Antineoplastic agent. Anthracycline antibiotic isolated from Actinomadura carminata. $[\alpha]_D^{20}$ = 289°; λ_m = 236, 255, 462, 478, 492 nm; soluble in H$_2$O, MeOH; insoluble in organic solvents; LD$_{50}$ (mus orl) = 7.3 mg/kg, (mus iv) = 1.3 mg/kg, (mus sc) = 3.7 mg/kg.

75 Carzelesin
119813-10-4

$C_{41}H_{37}ClN_6O_5$
(S)-N-[2-[[1-(Chloromethyl)-1,6-dihydro-8-methyl-5-[[(phenylamino)carbonyl]-oxy]benzo[1,2-b;4,3-b']dipyrrol-3(2H)-

yl]carbonyl]-1H-indol-5-yl]-6-diethylamino)-2-benzofuran-carboxamide.
U-80244. Antineoplastic agent.

76   CeeNU
13010-47-4   5594   235-859-2

$C_9H_{16}ClN_3O_2$
N-(2-Chloroethyl)-N'-cyclohexyl-N-nitrosourea.
Lomustine; CCNU; RB-1509; Belustine; Cecenu; CiNU; NSC-79037. Antineoplastic agent. mp= 90°; insoluble in H_2O, soluble in organic solvents; LD_{50} (mus orl) = 51 mg/kg, (mus ip) = 56 mg/kg, (mus sc) = 61 mg/kg. Bristol-Myers Oncology.

77   Cemadotin
159776-69-9

$C_{35}H_{56}N_6O_5$
N,N-Dimethyl-L-valyl-L-valyl-N-methyl-L-valyl-L-prolyl-N-benzyl-L-prolinamide.
Potential antitumor agent.

78   Chlorambucil
305-03-3   2116

$C_{14}H_{19}Cl_2NO_2$
4-[Bis(2-chloroethyl)amino]-benzenebutanoic acid.
Leukeran   Tablets;   4-[p-[bis(2-chloro-ethyl)amino]phenyl]butyric acid; Ambo-

chlorin;   Leukeran;   chloraminophene; CB-1348;   NSC-3088.   Antineoplastic agent. A   proprietary   formulation of chlorambucil; for treatment of chronic lymphocytic   leukemia,   Hodgkins disease, certain forms of non-Hodgkins lymphoma,   Walderstroms   macro-globuliremia   and   advanced   ovarian adenocarcinoma. mp = 64-66°; soluble in Et_2O,   alcohol, $CHCl_3$, Me_2OH; insoluble in H_2O; LD_{50} (rat ip) = 17.7 mg/kg. Glaxo Wellcome Inc.

79   Chlornaphazine
494-03-1   2157

$C_{14}H_{15}Cl_2N$
N,N-Bis(2-chloroethyl)-2-naphthylamine.
CB-1048; R-48; Cloronaftina; Erysan; NSC-62209. Antineoplastic agent. mp = 54°; bp = 210°; poorly soluble in H_2O (< 0.1 mg/l), more soluble in organic solvents.

80   Chromomycin A3
7059-24-7   2295

$C_{57}H_{82}O_{26}$
3β-O-(4-O-Acetyl-2,6-dideoxy-3-C-methyl-α-L-arabino-hexopyranosyl)-7-methylolivomycin D.

Aburamycin B; Chromomycin; Toyo-mycin; NSC-58514. Antineoplastic agent. mp = 185° (dec); $[\alpha]_D^{23}$ = -55° (EtOH); λ_m = 230, 281, 304, 318, 330, 412 nm (log ε 4.39, 4.72, 3.85, 3.92, 3.84, 4.07); LD_{50} (mus iv) = 1.85 mg/kg, (mus ip) = 1.7 mg/kg.

81 Ciaftalan Zinc
14320-04-8

$C_{32}H_{16}N_8Zn$
(SP-4-1)-[Phthalocyaninato(2-)-
$N^{29},N^{30},N^{31},N^{32}$]zinc.
Used in photodynamic therapeutic treatment of cancer.

82 Cirolemycin
11056-12-5
U-12241. Antineoplastic antibiotic produced by Streptomyces bellus.

83 Cisplatin
15663-27-1   2378   239-733-8

$Cl_2H_6N_2Pt$
cis-Diamminedichloroplatinum.
cis-diamminedichloroplatinum; cis-platinum II; cis-DDP; CACP; CPDC; DDP; Briplatin; Cismaplat; Cisplatyl; Citoplatino; Lederplatin; Neoplatin; Platamine; Platinex; Platiblastin; Platinol; Platinoxan; Platistin; Platosin; Rand; NSC-119875. Antineoplastic agent. mp = 270° (dec); soluble in H_2O (253 mg/100g), insoluble in organic solvents; LD_{50} (gpg ip) = 9.7 mg/kg. Lederle Labs.

84 Cladribine
4291-63-8   2397

$C_{10}H_{12}ClN_5O_3$
2-Chloro-2'-deoxyadenosine.
leustatin; RWJ-26251; NSC-105014; cladribine; 2-CdA; CldAdo. Antineoplastic agent. mp = 220° (softens); $[\alpha]_D^{25}$ = -18.8° (DMF, c = 1.0); λ_m = 265 nm (0.1n NaOH), 265 nm (0.1N HCl). Ortho Biotech Inc.

85 Clanfenur
51213-99-1

$C_{16}H_{15}ClFN_3O_2$
1-(p-Chlorophenyl)-3-(6-fluoro-N,N-dimethylanthraniloyl)urea.
Antineoplastic.

86 Condyline
518-28-5   7704   208-250-4

$C_{22}H_{22}O_8$
[5R-(5α,5aβ,8aα,9α)]-5,8,8a,9-
Tetrahydro-9-hydroxy-5-(3,4,5-
trimethoxyphenyl)-furo[3',4':6,7]-
naphtho[2,3-d]-1,3-dioxol-6(5aH)-one.
Bisoprolol; podofilox; podophyllotoxin; NSC-24818. mp = 114-118°, 183-184°;

$[\alpha]_D^{20}$ = -132.7° (CHCl$_3$); soluble in H$_2$O (120 mg/l), more soluble in organic solvents; LD$_{50}$ (rat iv) = 8.7 mg/kg, (rat ip) = 15 mg/kg. *E. Merck.*

87   Crisnatol
96389-68-3

C$_{23}$H$_{23}$NO$_2$
2-[(6-Chrysenylmethyl)amino]-2-methyl-1,3-propanediol.
BW-A770U. Antineoplastic agent. *Glaxo Wellcome Inc.*

88   Crisnatol Mesylate
96389-69-4

C$_{24}$H$_{27}$NO$_5$S
2-[(6-Chrysenylmethyl)amino]-2-methyl 1,3-propanediol methanesulfonate (salt).
BW-A770U mesylate. Antineoplastic agent. *Glaxo Wellcome Inc.*

89   Cyclophosphamide
50-18-0   2816   200-015-4

C$_7$H$_{15}$Cl$_2$N$_2$O$_2$P
(Bis(chloro-2-ethyl)amino)-2-tetrahydro-3,4,5,6-oxazaphosphorine-1,3,2-oxide-2 hydrate.
ASTA-B-518;   Clafen;   Claphene;

Cyclophosphamid; Cyclophosphamide; Cyclophosphamidum; Cyclophosphan; Cyclophosphane; Cyclostin; Cytophosphan; Cytoxan; NSC-26271; CB-4564; CP; CPA; CTX; CY; Endoxan; Endoxan R; Endoxan-Asta; Endoxana; Endoxanal; Endoxane; Enduxan; Genoxal; Hexadrin; Mitoxan; Neosar; NCI-C04900; Procytox; Semdoxan; Sendoxan; Senduxan; SK 20501; Zyklophosphamid. Antineoplastic agent. mp = 41-45°; soluble in H$_2$O (40 g/l), less soluble in oganic solvents; LD$_{50}$ (rat orl) = 94 mg/kg. *Pharmacia & Upjohn, Inc.; Bristol-Myers Oncology.*

90   Cyclophosphamide, Hydrated
6055-19-2   2816

C$_7$H$_{15}$Cl$_2$N$_2$O$_2$P.H$_2$O
N,N-bis(2-Chloroethyl)tetrahydro-2H-1,3,2-oxazaphosphorin-2-amine 2-oxide.
2-[bis(2-chloroethyl)amino]tetrahydro-2H-1,3,2-oxazophosphorine 2-oxide; 1-bis-(2-chloroethyl)amino-1-oxa-2-aza-5-oxaphosphoridin; B 518; Cycloblastin; Cyclostin; Endoxan; Procytox; Sendoxan; Cytoxan; NSC-26271. Antineoplastic agent. mp = 41-45°; soluble in H$_2$O (40 g/l), less soluble in oganic solvents; LD$_{50}$ (rat orl) = 94 mg/kg. *Degussa AG.*

91   Cytadren
125-84-8   460   204-756-4

C$_{13}$H$_{16}$N$_2$O$_2$
3-(4-Aminophenyl)-3-ethyl-2,6-piperidinedione.
aminoglutethimide;   p-Aminoglutethimide; Ba-16038; Elipten; NSC-330915; 2-(p-Aminophenyl)-2-ethylglutarimide; 3-

(4-aminophenyl)-3-ethyl-2,6-piperidine-dione. Antineoplastic agent. mp = 149-150°; insoluble in H_2O, soluble in organic solvents. *Ciba-Geigy Corp.*

92 Cytarabine
147-94-4   2853   205-705-9

$C_9H_{13}N_3O_5$
4-Amino-1-β-D-arabinofuranosyl-2(1H)-pyrimidinone.
1-β-D-arabinofuranosylcytosine; β-cytosine arabino-side; CHX-3311; U-19920; Alexan; Arabitin; Aracytidine; Aracytine; Ara-C; Cytosar; Cytosar U; Erpalfa; Iretin; Udicil; NSC-287459. Antineoplastic agent and antiviral agent. mp = 212-213°; $[\alpha]_D^{23}$ = 158° (c = 0.5, H_2O); λ_m = 281, 212.5 nm (ε 13171, 10230, pH 2). *Ciba-Geigy Corp.*

93 Cytosar-U
147-94-4   2853   205-705-9

$C_9H_{13}N_3O_5$
4-Amino-1-β-D-arabinofuranosyl-2(1H)-pyrimidinone.
1-β-D-arabinofuranosylcytosine; β-cytosine arabino-side; CHX-3311; U-19920; Alexan; Arabitin; Aracytidine; Aracytine; Ara-C; Cytosar; Cytosar U; Erpalfa; Iretin; Udicil; NSC-287459. Antineoplastic agent and antiviral agent. mp = 212-213°; $[\alpha]_D^{23}$ = 158° (c = 0.5, H_2O); λ_m = 281, 212.5 nm (ε 13171, 10230, pH 2). *Ciba-Geigy Corp.*

94 Dacarbazine
4342-03-4   2866   224-396-1

$C_6H_{10}N_6O$
5-(3,3-Dimethyl-1-triazenyl)-1H-imidazole-4-carboxamide.
(Dimethyltriazeno)imidazolecarboxamide; Dacarbazine; Deticene; NSC-45388; dimethyltriazenoimidazolecarboxamide; DIC; DTIC; DTIC-Dome; DTIE; Imidazole carboxamide; ICDMT; ICDT; NCI-C04717. Antineoplastic agent. Dec (explosive) 250-255°; λ_m = 237 nm (ε 11200 pH 7); insoluble in H_2O (10 mg/100 ml), organic solvents; LD_{50} (rat orl) = 2147 mg/kg. *Bayer Corp., Pharmaceutical Div.*

95 Dactinomycin
50-76-0   2867

$C_{62}H_{86}N_{12}O_{16}$
Specific stereoisomer of N,N'-[(2-amino-4,6-dimethyl-3-oxo-3H-phenoxazine-1,9-diyl)bis[carbonylimino[2-hydroxy-propylidene)carbonyliminoisobutylidene carbonyl-1,2-pyrrolidinediylcarbonyl-(methylimino)methylenecarbonyl]]bis[N-methyl-L-valine] dilactone.
Actinomycin 7; actinomycindioic D acid dilactone; NSC-3053; Actactinomycin A

IV; Actinomycin AIV; Actinomycin D; Actinomycin IV; Actinomycin X 1; actinomycin[thr-val-pro-sar-meval]; Cosmegen; C1; Dactinomycin; Dactinomycin D; Dilactone actinomycin D acid; Dilactone actinomycindioic D acid; HBF-386; Lyovac cosmegen; meractinomycin; NCI-C04682; Oncostatin K. Antineoplastic agent. Antibiotic from *Streptomyces parvullus*. mp = 241-243° (dec); $[\alpha]_D^{28}$ = -315° (MeOH, c = 0.25); λ_m = 244, 441 nm ($A_{1\ cm}^{1\%}$ 281, 206); soluble in organic solvents; light sensitive; LD_{50} (mus orl) = 13.0 mg/kg, (rat orl) = 7.2 mg/kg. *Merck & Co., Inc.*

96   Datelliptium Chloride
105118-14-7

$C_{23}H_{28}ClN_3O$
2-[2-(Diethylamino)ethyl]-9-hydroxy-5,11-dimethyl-6H-pyrido[4,3-b]-carbazolium chloride.
Antineoplastic.

97   Daunorubicin
20830-81-3   2890

$C_{27}H_{29}NO_{10}$
8-Acetyl-10-[(3-amino-2,3,6-trideoxy-alpha-L-lyxo-hexopyranosyl)oxy]-7,8,9,10-tetrahydro-6,8,11-trihydroxy-1-methoxy-,(8S-cis)-5,12-naphthacene-dione.
Cerubidine; daunoblastin; daunomycin; FI-6339; leukaemomycin C; RP-13057; rubidomycin. Antineoplastic agent. Anthracine antibiotic from *Streptomyces coeruleorubidus*. mp = 208-209°; LD_{50} (mus iv) = 20 mg/kg, (mis ip) = 5 mg/kg,

(rat iv) = 13 mg/kg, (rat ip) = 8 mg/kg. *Rhône-Poulenc Rorer Pharmaceuticals Inc.; Wyeth-Ayerst Labs.*

98   Daunorubicin Hydrochloride
23541-50-6   2890

$C_{27}H_{30}ClNO_{10}$
8-Acetyl-10-[(3-amino-2,3,6-trideoxy-alpha-L-lyxo-hexopyranosyl)oxy]-7,8,9,10-tetrahydro-6,8,11-trihydroxy-1-methoxy-,(8S-cis)-5,12-naphthacene-dione monohydrochloride.
Cerubidine; daunoblastin; daunomycin hydrochloride; daunorubicin HCL; NSC-82151; NDC-0082-4155; Ondena; Rubidomycin hydrochloride; RP-13057 hydrochloride; Daunoblastina. Antineoplastic agent. mp = 188-190° (dec); $[\alpha]_D^{20}$ = 248° (MeOH, c = 0.05-0.10); soluble in H_2O, polar organic solvents; insoluble in non-polar organic solvents; λ_m = 234, 252, 290, 480, 495, 532 nm ($E_{1\ cm}^{1\%}$ = 665 462, 153, 214, 218, 112, MeOH); LD_{50} (mus iv)= 26 mg/kg. *Rhône-Poulenc Rorer Pharmaceuticals Inc.; Wyeth-Ayerst Labs.*

99   Decitabine
2353-33-5

$C_8H_{12}N_4O_4$
4-Amino-1-(2-deoxy-β-D-erythro-pentofuranosyl)-3,5-triazin-2(1H)-one.
5-Aza-2'-deoxycytidine; NSC-127716; Decitabine. Antineoplastic agent. *Pharmachemie U.S.A., Inc.*

100   Defosfamide
3733-81-1   2917

$C_9H_{20}Cl_3N_2O_3P$
N,N-Bis(2-chloroethyl)-N'-(3-hydroxy-propyl)phosphorodiamidic acid
2-chloroethyl ester.
B-612; B 612-Asta; Defosfamid; Defosfamide; Desmofosfamide; Desmophosphamidum; Mitarson; NSC-40627. Antineoplastic agent. Liquid; sg = 1.3675; insoluble in H_2O, soluble in organic solvents.

101   Demecolcine
477-30-5   2938

$C_{21}H_{25}NO_5$
Deacetyl-N-methylcolchicine.
C-12669; Alkaloid H 3, from Colchicum autumnale; C-12669; Ciba 12669 A; Colcemide; Colchamine; NSC-3096; N-deacetyl-N-methylcolchicine; Kolchamin; Kolkamin; Omaine; Reichstein's F; Santavy's substance F; Substance F. Antineoplastic agent. mp = 186°; $[\alpha]_D^{20}$ = -129.0° ($CHCl_3$ c = 1); λ_m = 245 355 nm (log ε 4.55 4.24 EtOH); soluble in acid solutions, organic solvents.

102   Detorubicin
66211-92-5

$C_{33}H_{39}NO_{14}$
2-(Diethyl acetal) glyoxylic acid 3^2 ester doxorubicin b.
Antineoplastic.

103   Dexormaplatin
96392-96-0
$C_6H_{14}Cl_4N_2Pt$
(+)-trans-Tetrachloro(1,2-cyclohexanediamine)platinum.
U-78938. Antineoplastic agent. *Pharmacia & Upjohn, Inc.*

104   Dexrazoxane
24584-09-6   8295

$C_{11}H_{16}N_4O_4$
4,4'-(1-Methyl-1,2-ethanediyl)bis-2,6-piperazinedione.
ICI-59118; ICRF-159; Razoxin; Zinecard; ADR-529; NSC-129943; Cardioxane [as (+) hydrochloride]; Eucardion [as (+) hydrochloride]. Cardioprotectant. The (+) isomer is a cardioprotectant. The (±) form is an antineoplastic. [(+) isomer]: mp = 193°; $[\alpha]_D$ = 11.35° (DMF c = 5); soluble in H_2O (10 mg/ml), organic solvents. *Pharmacia & Upjohn, Inc.*

105   Dezaguanine
41729-52-6

C₆H₆N₄O
6-Amino-1,5-dihydro-4H-imidazo-
[4,5-c]pyridin-4-one.
CI-908; ICN-4221; NSC-261726. Antineoplastic agent. *Parke-Davis*.

106   Dezaguanine Mesylate
87434-82-0

CH₃SO₃H

C₇H₁₀N₄O₄S
6-Amino-1,5-dihydro-4H-imidazo-
[4,5-c]pyridin-4-one methanesulfonate.
CI-908 mesylate; PD-90695-73. Antineoplastic agent. *Parke-Davis*.

107   Diaziquone
57998-68-2   3044

C₁₆H₂₀N₄O₆
[2,5-Bis(1-aziridinyl)-3,6-dioxo-1,4-
cyclohexadiene-1,4-diyl]bis-carbamic
acid diethyl ester.
AZQ; CI-904; NSC-182986. Antineoplastic agent. mp = 230° (dec); λₘ =
340 nm (log ε 4.17); soluble in H₂O (0.5
mg/ml); LD₅₀ (mus iv) = 30.9 mg/m².
Parke-Davis.

108   Dinaline
58338-59-3

C₁₃H₁₃N₃O
2',4-Diaminobenzanilide.
Antineoplastic.

109   Ditercalinium Chloride
74517-42-3

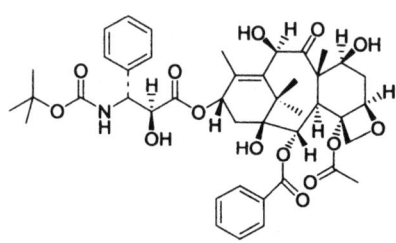

C₄₆H₅₀Cl₂N₆O₂
2,2'-([4,4'-Bipiperidine]-1,1'-diyl-
diethylene)bis[10-methoxy-7H-
pyrido[4,3-c]cabrazolium] dichloride.
Antineoplastic.

110   Docetaxel
148408-66-6

C₄₃H₅₃NO₁₄.3H₂O
[2aR-[2aα,4β,4aβ,6β,9α(αR*,βS*),11α,
12α,12aα,12bα]]-β-12b-(Acetyloxy)-12-
(benzoyloxy)-2a,3,4,4a,5,6,9,10,11,
12,12a,12b-dodecahydro-4,6,11-tri-
hydroxy-4a,8,13,13-tetramethyl-5-oxo-
7,11-methano-1H-cyclodeca[3,4]benz-
[1,2-b]oxet-9-yles [[(1,1-dimethyl-
ethoxy)carbonyl]amino]-α-hydroxy-
benzenepropanoic acid trihydrate.

RP-56976; taxotere. Antineoplastic agent. Binds to tubulin and inhibits depolymerization of microtubules. *Rhône-Poulenc Rorer Pharmaceuticals Inc.*

111 Docetaxel [anhydrous]
114977-28-5 3458

$C_{43}H_{53}NO_{14}$
[2aR-[2aα,4β,4aβ,6β,9α(αR*,βS*),11α,12α,12aα,12bα]]-β-12b-(Acetyloxy)-12-(benzoyloxy)-2a,3,4,4a,5,6,9,10,11,12,12a,12b-dodecahydro-4,6,11-trihydroxy-4a,8,13,13-tetramethyl-5-oxo-7,11-methano-1H-cyclodeca[3,4]benz-[1,2-b]oxet-9-yles [[(1,1-dimethyl-ethoxy)carbonyl]amino]-α-hydroxy-benzenepropanoic acid.
taxotere; docetaxel; N-debenzoyl-N-tert-butoxycarbonyl-10-deacetyl taxol. Antineoplastic agent. Binds to tubulin and inhibits depolymerization of microtubules. mp = 232°; $[\alpha]_D$ = -36° (EtOH c= 0.74); λ_m = 230, 275, 283 nm (ε 14800, 1730, 1670).

112 Doxifluridine
3094-09-5 3493

$C_9H_{11}FN_2O_5$
5'-Deoxy-4-fluorouridine.
5'-DFUR; 5'-dFUrd; Ro-21-9738; Flutron; Furtulon. Antineoplastic agent. mp = 189-190°, 186-188°, 192-193°;

$[\alpha]_D^{25}$ = 18.4° (H$_2$O c = 0.419); λ_m = 268-269 nm(ε 8550); LD$_{50}$ (mus iv 14 day) > 1000 mg/kg, (rat iv 14 day) > 2000 mg/kg, (mrat orl) = 3471 mg/kg, (frat orl) = 3390 mg/kg, (mmus orl) > 5000 mg/kg, (fmus orl) > 5000 mg/kg. *Hoffmann-LaRoche Inc.*

113 Doxorubicin
23214-92-8 3495

$C_{27}H_{29}NO_{11}$
α-3b-Glycoloyl-1,2,3,4,6,11-hexahydro-3,5,12-trihydroxy-10-methoxy-6,11-dioxo-1a-naphthacenyl 3-amino-2,3,6-trideoxy-L-lyxo-hexopyranoside.
adriblastina; FI-106. Antineoplastic agent. mp = 229-231°. *Farmitalia, Societa Farmaceutici.*

114 Doxorubicin Hydrochloride
25316-40-9 3495

$C_{27}H_{30}ClNO_{11}$
α-3b-Glycoloyl-1,2,3,4,6,11-hexahydro-3,5,12-trihydroxy-10-methoxy-6,11-dioxo-1a-naphthacenyl 3-amino-2,3,6-trideoxy-L-lyxo-hexopyranoside hydrochloride.
Adriacin; adriamycin hydrochloride; adriamycin hydrochloride (8Cl); Adriblastin; NSC-123127; Adriblastina; ADM hydrochloride; ADR; Doxorubicin; Doxorubicin hydrochloride; DOX HCl; FI 106; FI 6804; Hydroxydaunorubicin hydrochloride. Antineoplastic agent. mp = 204-205°; $[\alpha]_D^{20}$ = 248° (MeOH c= 0.1); λ_m = 233, 252, 288, 479, 496, 529 nm;

soluble in H_2O, polar organic solvents; LD_{50} (mus iv) = 21.1 mg/kg. *Farmitalia, Societa Farmaceutici.*

115   DTIC-Dome
4342-03-4　　　　2866　224-396-1

$C_6H_{10}N_6O$
5-(3,3-Dimethyl-1-triazenyl)-1H-imidazole-4-carboxamide.
Dacarbazine; Deticene; NSC-45388; Dimethyltriazenoimidazolecarboxamide; DIC; DTIC; DTIC-Dome; DTIE; Imidazole carboxamide; ICDMT; ICDT; NCI-C04717. Antineoplastic agent. Dec (explosive) 250-255°; λ_m = 223 nm (ε 7500 0.1N HCl), 237 nm (ε 11200 pH 7); insoluble in H_2O (10 mg/100 ml), organic solvents; LD_{50} (rat orl) = 2147 mg/kg. *Bayer Corp., Pharmaceutical Div.*

116   Duazomycin
1403-47-0
$C_8H_{11}N_3O_4$
N-Acetyl-6-diazo-5-oxo L-norleucine.
A-10270A; Acetyl-DON; Diazomycin A; Duazomycin (USAN); Duazomycin A; NSC-51097. Antineoplastic agent. An antibiotic from *Streptomyces ambofaciens.* *Pfizer Inc.*

117   Ecomustine
98383-18-7

$C_{10}H_{18}ClN_3O_6$
Methyl 3-[3-(2-chloroethyl)-3-nitroso-ureido]-2,3-dideoxy-α-D-arabinohexapyranoside.
Antineoplastic.

118   Edaravone
89-25-8　　　　　　　6809

$C_{10}H_{10}N_2O$
2,4-Dihydro-5-methyl-2-phenyl-3H-pyrazol-3-one.
NSC-12; NSC-2629; NSC-26139; C.I. Developer 1; Developer Z; Methyl-phenylpyrazolone; Norphenazone; NCI-C03952. Antineoplastic agent. Used in treatment of stroke. mp = 129-130°; bp_{265} = 287°. *Pfalz & Bauer.*

119   Edatrexate
80576-83-6　　　　　　　3553

$C_{22}H_{25}N_7O_5$
N-[4-[1-[(2,4-Diamino-6-pteridinyl)-methyl]propyl]benzoyl]-L-glutamic acid.
10-Ethyl-10-dezazaminopterin; Psyllium; NSC-626715; 10-EdAM; CGP-30694. Antineoplastic agent. λ_m = 255, 370 nm (ε 30731, 7582 pH 12). *Ciba-Geigy Corp.*

120   Edelfosine
70641-51-9

$C_{27}H_{58}NO_6P$
(±)-2-Methoxy-3-(octadecyloxy)propyl hydrogen phosphate choline hydroxide inner salt.
Antineoplastic.

121 Eflornithine
67037-37-0   3564

C$_6$H$_{12}$F$_2$N$_2$O$_2$
2-Difluoromethyl-L-ornithine.
Antineoplastic agent. A proprietary preparation of thiamine hydrochloride, nicotinamide, tincture of gentian and caffeine hydrate; a tonic. *Marion Merrell Dow Inc.*

122 Eflornithine Hydrochloride
96020-91-6   3564

C$_6$H$_{13}$ClF$_2$N$_2$O$_2$.H$_2$O
2-Difluoromethyl-L-ornithine monohydrochloride monohydrate.
Ornidyl; MDL-71782A. Antineoplastic agent. mp = 183°. *Marion Merrell Dow Inc.*

123 Efudex
51-21-8   4219   200-085-6

C$_4$H$_3$FN$_2$O$_2$
5-Fluoro-2,4(1H,3H)-Pyrimidinedione.
Fluorouracil; FU; 5-FU; Adrucil; Efudex; Fluoroplex; Ro-2-9757; Arumel; Carzonal; Effluderm (free base); Efudix; Fluoroblastin; Fluracil; Fluri; Fluril; Kecimeton; Timazin; U-8953; Ulup; 5-

Ftouracyl; efurix; fluracilum; ftoruracil; queroplex; NSC-19893. Antineoplastic agent. mp = 282-283° (dec); λ_m = 265-266 nm (ϵ 7070 0.1N HCl); insoluble in H$_2$O; LD$_{50}$ (rat orl) = 230 mg/kg. *Hoffmann-LaRoche Inc.*

124 Elacridar
143664-11-3

C$_{34}$H$_{33}$N$_3$O$_5$
N-[4-(2-(3,4-Dihydro-6,7-dimethoxy-2(1h)-isoquinolyl)ethyl]phenyl]-9,10-dihydro-5-methoxy-9-oxo-4-acridinecarboxamide.
Antineoplastic agent (adjunct). *Glaxo Wellcome Inc.*

125 Elacridar Hydrochloride
143851-98-3

C$_{34}$H$_{34}$ClN$_3$O$_5$
N-[4-(2-(3,4-Dihydro-6,7-dimethoxy-2(1h)-isoquinolyl)ethyl]phenyl]-9,10-dihydro-5-methoxy-9-oxo-4-acridinecarboxamide hydrochloride.
GF-120918A. Antineoplastic agent (adjunct). *Glaxo Wellcome Inc.*

126   Eldisine
59917-39-4   10125   261-984-7

$C_{43}H_{57}N_5O_{11}S$
3-(Aminocarbonyl)-O^4-deacetyl-3-
de(methoxycarbonyl)sulfate (1:1) (salt).
vindesine sulfate; LY-099094; NSC-
245467. Antineoplastic agent. mp >
250°; LD_{50} (mus iv) = 6.3 mg/kg, (rat iv) =
2.0 mg/kg, (mus ip) = 8.8 mg/kg. *Eli Lilly
& Co.*

127   Elliptinium Acetate
58337-35-2   3590

$C_{20}H_{20}N_2O_3$
9-Hydroxy-2,5,11-trimethyl-6H-
pyrido[4,3-b]carbazolium acetate.
Celiptium; 9-Hydroxy-2-methylellipti-
cinium acetate; Ellipticine analog;
H9M2E; NMHE; NSC-264137.
Antineoplastic agent.

128   Elmustine
60784-46-5

$C_5H_{10}ClN_3O_3$
1-(2-Chloroethyl)-3-(2-hydroxyethyl)-1-
nitrosourea.
Antineoplastic.

129   Elsamitrucin
97068-30-9

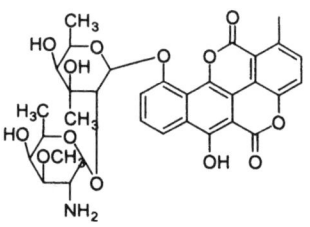

$C_{33}H_{35}NO_{13}$
10-[[2-O-(2-Amino-2,6-dideoxy-3-O-
methyl-α-D-galactopyranosyl)-6-deoxy-
3-C-methyl-β-D-galactopyranosyl]oxy]-6-
hydroxy-1-methyl-benzo[h][1]benzo-
pyrano[5,4,3-cde][1]benzopyran-5,12-
dione.
Chartreusin analog; Elsamicin; NSC-
369327. Antineoplastic agent. *Bristol-
Myers Squibb Pharmaceutical Res. and
Dev.*

130   Emcyt
52205-73-9   3749   257-735-7

$C_{23}H_{31}Cl_2NO_3$
Estra-1,3,5(10)-triene-3,17β-diol 3-[bis(2-
chloroethyl)carbamate].
Estracyt; Estradiol, [3-[bis(2-chloroethyl)-
carbamate]]dihydrogen phosphate (8CI);
Leo 299; NSC-89199; Estradiol 3-bis(2-
chloroethyl)carbamate; estra-1,3,5(10)-
triene-3,17β-diol   3-[N,N-bis-(2-chloro-
ethyl)carbamate]; Ro-21-8837. mp =
104-105°; $[\alpha]_D^{20}$ = 50° (dioxane); λ_m = 271,
277 nm. *Pharmacia & Upjohn, Inc.*

131 Emitefur

110690-43-2 3601

$C_{28}H_{19}FN_4O_8$
m-[[3-(Ethoxymethyl)-5-fluoro-3,6-dihydro-2,6-dioxo-1(2H)-pyrimidinyl]-carbonyl]benzoic acid 2-ester with 2,6-dihydroxynicotinonitrile benzoate.
Antineoplastic. mp = 162-164°; LD$_{50}$ (mus orl) > 5000 mg/kg, (frat orl) = 1850 mg/kg, (mrat orl) = 1934 mg/kg.

132 Endoxan

50-18-0 2816 200-015-4

$C_7H_{15}Cl_2N_2O_2P$
(Bis(chloro-2-ethyl)amino)-2-tetrahydro-3,4,5,6-oxazaphosphorine-1,3,2-oxide-2 hydrate.
ASTA-B-518; Clafen; Claphene; Cyclophosphamid; Cyclophosphamide; Cyclophosphamidum; Cyclophosphan; Cyclophosphane; Cyclostin; Cytophosphan; Cytoxan; NSC-26271; CB-4564; CP; CPA; CTX; CY; Endoxan; Endoxan R; Endoxan-Asta; Endoxana; Endoxanal; Endoxane; Enduxan; Genoxal; Hexadrin; Mitoxan; Neosar; NCI-C04900; Procytox; Semdoxan; Sendoxan; Senduxan; SK-20501; Zyklophosphamid. Antineoplastic agent. mp = 41-45°; soluble in H$_2$O (40 g/l), less soluble in oganic solvents; LD$_{50}$ (rat orl) = 94 mg/kg. *Pharmacia & Upjohn, Inc.; Bristol-Myers Oncology.*

133 Eniluracil

59989-18-3

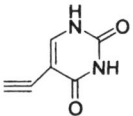

$C_6H_4N_2O_2$
5-Ethynyl-2,4(1H,3H)-pyrimidinedione.
776C85. Antineoplastic agent (adjunct).
Glaxo Wellcome Inc.

134 Enloplatin

111523-41-2

$C_{13}H_{22}N_2O_5Pt$
(SP-4-2)-[1,1-Cyclobutanedicarboxylato-(2-)](tetrahydro-4H-pyran-4,4-dimethanamine-N,N') platinum.
CL-287110. Antineoplastic agent. *Lederle Labs.*

135 Enocitabine

55726-47-1 3624

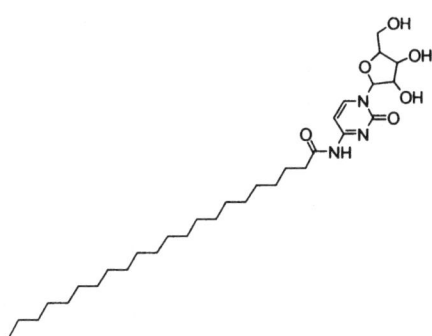

$C_{31}H_{55}N_3O_6$
N-(1-β-D-Arabinofuranosyl-1,2-dihydro-2-oxo-4-pyrimidinyl)docosanamide.
Antineoplastic agent. mp = 141-142°; [α]$_D$ = 70° (c = 1, THF); λ$_m$ = 216, 248, 303 nm (ε 16400, 15200, 8200 iPrOH).

136   Enpromate
10087-89-5

$C_{22}H_{23}NO_2$
1,1-Diphenyl-2-propynyl
cyclohexancarbamate.
59156;   NSC-112682.   Antineoplastic
agent. *Eli Lilly & Co.*

137   Epipropidine
5696-17-3

$C_{16}H_{28}N_2O_2$
1,1'-Bis(2,3-epoxypropyl)-4,4'-
bipiperidine.
Epipropidine; Eponate; Epoxypropidine;
Lilly 28002; NSC-56308. Antineoplastic
agent. *Eli Lilly & Co.*

138   Epirubicin
56420-45-2   3660

$C_{27}H_{29}NO_{11}$
(1S,3S)-Glycoloyl-1,2,3,4,6,11-
hexahydro-3,5,12-trihydroxy-10-
methoxy-6,11-dioxo-1-naphthacenyl
3-amino-2,3,6-trideoxy-α-L-arabino
hexopyranoside.

pidorubicin; 4'-epidoxorubicin; 4'-epi-
DX; IMI-28. Antineoplastic agent. Analog
of   the   anthracycline   antibiotic
doxorubicin differing only in the position
of the C_4 hydroxyl of the sugar moiety.
Farmitalia Carlo Erba SpA.

139   Epirubicin Hydrochloride
56390-09-1   3660

$C_{27}H_{30}ClNO_{11}$
(1S,3S)-Glycoloyl-1,2,3,4,6,11-
hexahydro-3,5,12-trihydroxy-10-
methoxy-6,11-dioxo-1-naphthacenyl   3-
amino-2,3,6-trideoxy-α-L-arabino
hexopyranoside hydrochloride.
Farmorubicin;   Pharmorubicin.
Antineoplastic agent. Analog of the
anthracycline   antibiotic   doxorubicin
differing only in the position of the C_4
hydroxyl of the sugar moiety. mp = 185°
(dec); $[\alpha]_D^{20} = 274°$ (MeOH c = 0.01).
Farmitalia Carlo Erba SpA.

140   Erbulozole
124784-31-2

$C_{24}H_{27}N_3O_5S$
Ethyl (±)-cis-p-[[[2-(imidazol-1-ylmethyl)-
2-(p-methoxyphenyl)-1,3-dioxolan-4-
yl]methyl]thio]carbanilate.
Antineoplastic agent (adjunct). *Janssen
Pharmaceutical Inc.*

141   Esorubicin
63521-85-7

$C_{27}H_{29}NO_{10}$
(2S-(2α(8R*,10R*),4β,6β))-10-[(4-
Aminotetrahydro-6-methyl-2H-pyran-2-
yl)oxy]-7,8,9,10-tetrahydro-6,8,11-
trihydroxy-8-(hydroxyacetyl)-1-methoxy-
5,12-naphthacenedione.
deoxydoxorubicin. Antineoplastic agent.
Farmitalia Carlo Erba SpA.

142   Esorubicin Hydrochloride
63950-06-1

$C_{27}H_{30}ClNO_{10}$
(2S-(2α(8R*,10R*),4β,6β))-10-[(4-
Aminotetrahydro-6-methyl-2H-pyran-2-
yl)oxy]-7,8,9,10-tetrahydro-6,8,11-
trihydroxy-8-(hydroxyacetyl)-1-methoxy-
5,12-naphthacenedione hydrochloride.
4'-deoxydoxorubicin   hydrochloride;
escorubicin hydrochloride; IMI 58 ; NSC-
267469. Antineoplastic agent. *Farmitalia
Carlo Erba SpA.*

143   Estramustine
2998-57-4   3749

$C_{23}H_{31}Cl_2NO_3$

Estradiol 3-[bis(2-chloroethyl)carbamate].
Ro-22-2296/000; Leo 275; NSC-89201.
Antineoplastic agent. mp = 104-105°;
$[α]_D^{20} = 50°$ (dioxane); $λ_m$ = 271, 277 nm
(EtOH). *Hoffmann-LaRoche Inc.*

144   Estramustine Phosphate
52205-73-9   3749
$C_{23}H_{31}Cl_2NO_3$
Estra-1,3,5(10)-triene-3,17β-diol 3-[bis(2-
chloroethyl)carbamate].
Emcyt; NSC-89199; Estradiol 3-bis(2-
chloroethyl)carbamate;   estra-
1,3,5(10)triene-3,17β-diol 3-[N,N-bis-(2-
chloroethyl)carbamate];   Ro-21-8837.
Antineoplastic. mp = 155°; $[α]_D^{20} = 30°$
(dioxane); soluble in H_2O. *Hoffmann-
LaRoche Inc.*

145   Estramustine Phosphate Sodium
52205-73-9   3749   257-735-7
$C_{23}H_{30}Cl_2NNa_2O_6P$
Estradiol 3-[bis(2-chloroethyl)carbamate]
17-(dihydrogen   phosphate)   disodium
salt.
Ro-21-8837/001;   Emcyt;   NSC-89199.
Antineoplastic agent. mp = 155°; $[α]^{20}ks_D$
= 30° (dioxane); soluble in H_2O.
Hoffmann-LaRoche Inc.

146   Etoglucid
1954-28-5   3926   217-784-7

$C_{12}H_{22}O_6$
1,2:15,16-Diepoxy-4,7,10,13-
tetraoxahexadecane.
ICI-32865; ethoglucid; Ayerst 62013;
Diglycidyltriethylene   glycol;   Epodyl;
Ethoglucid; Etoglucid; Etoglucide; NSC-
80439; ICI-32865; Oxirane, 2,2'-(2,5,8,
11-tetraoxadodecane-1,12-diyl)bis-;
Triethylene   glycol   diglycidyl   ether;
Triethylene glycol, bis(2,3-epoxypropyl)
ether; TDE. Antineoplastic agent. mp = -
15°; $bp_{0.005}$ = 140°; d^{20} = 1.1312. *ICI.*

147 Etoposide
33419-42-0   3931

$C_{29}H_{32}O_{13}$
[5R-[5α,5aβ,8aα,9β(R*)]]-9-[(4,6-O-
Ethylidene-β-D-glucopyranosyl)oxy]-
5,8,8a,9-tetrahydro-5-(4-hydroxy-3,5-
dimethoxyphenyl)-furo[3',4':6,7]-
naphtho[2,3-d]-1,3-dioxol-6(5aH)-one.
Toposar; VePesid; VP-16-213; NSC-
141540; Demethy-epipodophylotoxin,
ethylidene glucoside; Epipodophyllotoxin VP-16213; Etoposide; EPE;
etoposide; Vepesid; Vepesid J; VP-16-
213; VP-16. Antineoplastic agent. mp =
236-251°; $[α]_D^{20}$ = -110.5° (CHCl$_3$ c = 0.6);
$λ_m$ = 283 nm (ε 4245 MeOH). Bristol-
Myers Oncology.

148 Etoposide Phosphate
117091-64-2

$C_{29}H_{33}O_{16}P$
[5R-[5α,5aβ,8aα,9β(R*)]]-5-[3,5-
Dimethoxy-4-(phosphonooxy)phenyl]-9-
[(4,6-O-ethylidene-β-D-glucopyranosyl)-
oxy]-5,8,8a,9-tetrahydro-furo[3',4':6,7]-
naphtho[2,3-d]-1,3-dioxol-6(5aH)-one.

BMY-40481. Antineoplastic agent.
Bristol-Myers Squibb Pharmaceutical Res.
and Dev.

149 Etoprine
18588-57-3

$C_{12}H_{12}Cl_2N_4$
2,4-Diamino-5-(3,4-dichlorophenyl)-6-
ethylpyrimidine.
Ethodichlorophen; NSC-3062. Antineoplastic agent.

150 Fadrozole
102676-47-1   3969

$C_{14}H_{13}N_3$
(±)-p-(5,6,7,8-Tetrahydroimidazo[1,5-
a]pyridin-5-yl)benzonitrile.
Antineoplastic agent. mp = 117-118°.
Ciba-Geigy Corp.

151 Fadrozole Hydrochloride
102676-96-0   3969

$C_{14}H_{14}ClN_3$
(±)-p-(5,6,7,8-Tetrahydroimidazo[1,5-a]-
pyridin-5-yl)benzonitrile
monohydrochloride.
CGS-16949A. Antineoplastic agent. mp
= 231-233°; soluble in H$_2$O. Ciba-Geigy
Corp.

152 Fazarabine
65886-71-7

$C_8H_{12}N_4O_5$
4-Amino-1-β-D-arabinofuranosyl-s-triazin-2(1H)-one.
ara-AC; 5-azacytosine arabinoside; Kymarabine; NSC-281272. Antineoplastic agent. Canine contagious hepatitis vaccine.

153 Fenretinide
65646-68-6   4040

$C_{26}H_{33}NO_2$
N-(4-Hydroxyphenyl)retinamide.
all-trans-4'-hydroxyretinanilide.
Antineoplastic agent. mp = 173-175°, 162-163°, 178-181°; λ_m = 370 nm (ε 44500 $CHCl_3$), λ_m = 362 nm (ε 47900 MeOH). *McNeil Pharmaceutical.*

154 Floxuridine
50-91-9   4148

$C_9H_{11}FN_2O_5$
2'-Deoxy-5-fluorouridine.
FUDR; NSC-26740. Antiviral and antineoplastic agent. mp = 150-151°; λ_m = 268 nm (ε 7570, pH 7.2), 270 nm (ε 6480, pH 14); $[\alpha]_D$ = 37° (H_2O), 48.6° (DMF). *Hoffmann-LaRoche Inc.*

155 Fludarabine
21679-14-1   4162

$C_{10}H_{12}FN_5O_4$
9-β-D-Arabinofuranosyl-2-fluoroadenine.
2-Fluoro Ara-A; NSC-118218; 2-Fluoroadenine arabinoside. Antineoplastic agent. mp = 260°; $[\alpha]_D^{25}$ = 17° (EtOH c = 0.1); λ_m = 262 nm (ε 13,200 pH 1), 261 nm (ε 14,800 pH 7), 262 nm (ε 15,000 pH 13); poorly soluble in H_2O, organic solvents. *Berlex Labs., Inc.*

156 Fludarabine Phosphate
75607-67-9   4162

$C_{10}H_{13}FN_5O_7P$
9-β-D-Arabinofuranosyl-2-fluoroadenine 5'-(dihydrogenphosphate).
2-F-ara-AMP; NSC-328002; Fludara; NSC-312887. Antineoplastic agent. Soluble in H_2O. *Berlex Labs., Inc.*

157 5-Fluorouracil
51-21-8   4219   200-085-6

$C_4H_3FN_2O_2$
5-Fluoro-2,4(1H,3H)-Pyrimidinedione.
Fluorouracil; FU; 5-FU; Adrucil; Efudex; Fluoroplex; Ro-2-9757; Arumel; Carzonal; Effluderm (free base); Efudix;

Fluoroblastin; Fluracil; Fluri; Fluril; Kecimeton; Timazin; U-8953; Ulup; 5-flourracyl; efurix; fluracilum; ftoruracil; queroplex; NSC-19893. Antineoplastic agent. mp = 282-283° (dec); λ_m = 265-266 nm (ε 7070 0.1N HCl); insoluble in H_2O; LD_{50} (rat orl) = 230 mg/kg.

158   Flurocitabine
40505-45-1

$C_9H_{10}FN_3O_4$
(2R,3R,3aS,9aR)-7-Fluoro-2,3,3a,9a-tetrahydro-3-hydroxy-6-imino-6H-furo[2',3':4,5]oxazolo[3,2-a]pyrimidine-2-methanol.
Ro-21-0702; AAFC; RN-37717-21-8; NSC-166641; Anhydro-arabinosyl-5-fluoro-cytosine; Cyclo cytidine, 5-fluoro-; Cyclo FC; 5-fluoro-O,2,2'-cyclocytidine; 5-F-Anhydro-ara-C hydrochloride. Antineoplastic agent. *Hoffmann-LaRoche Inc.*

159   Fosquidone
114517-02-1

$C_{28}H_{22}NO_6P$
Benzyl (±)-5,8,13,14-tetrahydro-14-methyl-8,13-dioxobenz[5,6]-isoindolo[2,1-b]isoquinolin-9-yl hydrogen phosphate.
GR-63178K. Antineoplastic agent. *Glaxo Wellcome, UK.*

160   Fostriecin
87810-56-8

$C_{19}H_{27}O_9P$
5,6-Dihydro-6-[3,4,6,13-tetrahydroxy-3-methyl-1,7,9,11-tridecatetraenyl]2H-pyran-2-one 4-(hydrogen phosphate). Antineoplastic agent. *Parke-Davis.*

161   Fostriecin Sodium
87860-39-7

$C_{19}H_{26}NaO_9P$
5,6-Dihydro-6-[3,4,6,13-tetrahydroxy-3-methyl-1,7,9,11-tridecatetraenyl]2H-pyran-2-one 4-(sodium hydrogen phosphate).
CI-920. Antineoplastic agent. *Parke-Davis.*

162   Fotemustine
92118-27-9   4285

$C_9H_{19}ClN_3O_5P$
(±)Diethyl [1-[3-(2-chloroethyl)-3-nitrosoureido]ethyl]phosphonate.
S-10036; Muphoran. Antineoplastic agent. mp = 85°.

163 Gallium Nitrate
13494-90-1   4364

GaN_3O_9
Gallium(III) nitrate (1:3), anhydrous.
gallium trinitrate; nitric acid, gallium salt; ganite; NSC-15200. Antineoplastic agent and calcium regulator. Inactive (NCI). Soluble in H_2O, EtOH, Et_2O; LD_{50} (mus iv) = 55 mg/kg, (rat iv) = 46 mg/kg, (rbt iv) = 43 mg/kg.

164 Galocitabine
124012-42-6

$C_{19}H_{22}FN_3O_8$
N-[1-(5-Deoxy-β-D-ribofuranosyl)-5-fluoro-1,2-dihydro-2-oxo-4-pyrimidinyl]-3,4,5-trimethoxybenzamide.
Antineoplastic.

165 Gemcitabine
95058-81-4   4392

$C_9H_{11}F_2N_3O_4$
2'-Deoxy-2',2'-difluorocytidine.
LY-188011;dFdC;   dFdCyd;   Gemzar;

NSC-613327. Antineoplastic agent. $[\alpha]_{365}$ = 425° (MeOH c = 0.96); λ_m = 234, 268 nm (ε 7810, 8560 EtOH); LD_{10} (rat iv) = 200 mg/m². Eli Lilly & Co.

166 Gemcitabine Hydrochloride
122111-03-9   4392

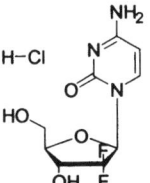

$C_9H_{12}ClF_2N_3O_4$
2'-Deoxy-2',2'-difluorocytidine hydrochloride.
mp = 287-292°; $[\alpha]_D$ = 48°; $[\alpha]_{365}$ = 257.9° (D_2O c = 1); λ_m = 232, 268 nm (ε 7960, 9360, H_2O).

167 Genoxal
50-18-0   2816   200-015-4

$C_7H_{15}Cl_2N_2O_2P$
(Bis(chloro-2-ethyl)amino)-2-tetrahydro-3,4 5,6-oxazaphosphorine-1,3,2-oxide-2 hydrate.
ASTA-B-518; Clafen; Claphene; Cyclophosphamid; Cyclophosphamide; Cyclophosphamidum; Cyclophosphan; Cyclophosphane; Cyclostin; Cytophosphan; Cytoxan; NSC-26271; CB-4564; CP; CPA; CTX; CY; Endoxan; Endoxan R; Endoxan-Asta; Endoxana; Endoxanal; Endoxane; Enduxan; Genoxal; Hexadrin; Mitoxan; Neosar; NCI-C04900; Procytox; Semdoxan; Sendoxan; Senduxan; SK-20501; Zyklophosphamid. Antineoplastic agent. mp = 41-45°; soluble in H_2O (40 g/l), less soluble in organic solvents; LD_{50} (rat orl) = 94 mg/kg. Pharmacia & Upjohn, Inc.; Bristol-Myers Oncology.

168   Gold Au-198
10043-49-9   4533
^{198}Au
Gold-198.
Colloidal gold (^{198}Au); Aurcoloid; Aureotrope; Auroscan-198. Antineoplastic agent. Radioactive agent (β- and γ-emitter) use as a diagnostic reagent in liver imaging. *Abbott Labs.; Bristol-Myers Squibb Pharmaceutical Res. and Dev; Mallinckrodt, Inc.*

169   Hexaprofen
24645-20-3

$C_{15}H_{20}O_2$
p-Cyclohexylhydratropic acid.
Reported to be anti-metastatic in Lewis lung tumors.

170   Holoxan
3778-73-2   4937   223-237-3

$C_7H_{15}Cl_2N_2O_2P$
3-(2-Chloroethyl)-2-[(2-chloroethyl)-amino]tetrahydro-2H-1,3,2-oxazaphosphorine 2-oxide.
Isophosphamide; Ifex; Iphosphamid; Isoendoxan; Cyfos; Holoxan; Mitoxana; Naxamide; A-4942; Asta-Z-4942; NSC-109724; Holoxan 1000; Ifosfamid; Iphosphamid; Isofosfamide; MJF-9325; Z4942. Antineoplastic agent. Cytostatic agent related to cyclophosphamide. mp = 39-41°; LD$_{50}$ (rat ip) = 160 mg/kg, 150 mg/kg. *Bristol-Myers Oncology.*

171   Honvan
522-40-7   4279   208-328-8

$C_{18}H_{22}O_8P_2$
α,α'-Diethyl-(E)-4,4'-stilbenediol bis(dihydrogen phosphate).
DESDP; diethylstilbesterol bisphosphate; diethylstilbestryl bisphosphate; fosfestrol; st52-asta; stilbestrol bisphosphate; stilphostrol; fosfesterol. Estrogen and antineoplastic agent. mp = 204-206° (dec); poorly soluble in H$_2$O. *Bayer Corp., Pharmaceutical Div.*

172   Hydroxyurea
127-07-1   4896   204-821-7

$CH_4N_2O_2$
N-(Aminocarbonyl)hydroxylamine.
Biosupressin; Hidrix; Hydrea; Hydreia; N-carbamoyl-hydroxylamine; hydroxylurea; hydroxyurea; NSC-32065; Hydura; Hydurea; HU; Litaler; Litalir; N-Hydroxyurea; NCI-C04831; Oncocarbide; Oxyurea; SK 22591; SQ-1089. mp = 133-136°; soluble in H$_2$O, EtOH. *Bristol-Myers Oncology.*

173   Idarubicin
58957-92-9   4931

$C_{26}H_{27}NO_9$
(7S-cis)-9-Acetyl-7-[(3-amino-2,3,6-trideoxy-α-L-lyxo-hexopyranosyl)oxy]-

7,8,9,10-tetrahydro-6,9,11-trihydroxy-
5,12-naphthacenedione.
Idarubicin; 4-DMD; 4-demethoxydauno-
rubicin; NSC-256439. Antineoplastic
agent. *Farmitalia Carlo Erba SpA.*

174 Idarubicin Hydrochloride
57852-57-0   4931

$C_{26}H_{28}ClNO_9$
(7S-cis)-9-Acetyl-7-[(3-amino-2,3,6-
trideoxy-α-L-lyxo-hexopyranosyl)oxy]-
7,8,9,10-tetrahydro-6,9,11-trihydroxy-
5,12-naphthacenedione hydrochloride.
4-demethoxydaunomycin hydrochloride;
Idarubicin hydrochloride; 4-DMD HCl;
NSC-256439; Idamycin; Zavedos.
Antineoplastic agent. mp = 183-185°,
172-174°; $[\alpha]_D^{20}$ = 205°, 188° (MeOH c =
0.1). *Farmitalia Carlo Erba SpA.*

175 Ifosfamide
3778-73-2   4937   223-237-3

$C_7H_{15}Cl_2N_2O_2P$
3-(2-Chloroethyl)-2-[(2-chloroethyl)-
amino]tetrahydro-2H-1,3,2-
oxazaphosphorine 2-oxide.
Isophosphamide; Ifex; Iphosphamid;
Isoendoxan; Cyfos; Holoxan; Mitoxana;
Naxamide; A-4942; Asta-Z-4942; NSC-
109724; Holoxan 1000; Ifosfamid;
Iphosphamid; Isofosfamide; MJF-9325; Z-
4942. Antineoplastic agent. mp = 39-41°;
LD_{50} (rat ip) = 150 mg/kg, 160 mg/kg.
Bristol-Myers Oncology.

176 Ilmofosine
89315-55-9

$C_{26}H_{56}NO_5PS$
(±)-3,5-Dioxa-9-thia-4-phospha-
pentacosan-1-aminium 4-hydroxy-7-
(methoxymethyl)-N,N,N-trimethyl
hydroxide inner salt 4-oxide.
BM-41440. *Boehringer Mannheim
GmbH.*

177 Imexon
59643-91-3

$C_4H_5N_3O$
4-Imino-1,3-diazabicyclo[3.1.0]-
hexan-2-one.
Antineoplastic.

178 Improsulfan
13425-98-4   4962

$C_8H_{19}NO_6S_2$
3,3'-Iminobis(1-propanol)
dimethanesulfonate.
Improsulfan tosylate; Improsulfan; NSC-
102627; Yoshi 864; Bis(3-
mesyloxypropyl)amine hydrochloride;
Compound 864; IPD; IPD hydrochloride.
mp = 94-95°; LD_{50} (rat iv) = 75 mg/kg.

179   Interferon alfa
74899-72-2
Alpha interferon.
Antineoplastic   agent   and
immunomodulator. Produced by human
lymphoblastoid cells induced with
Sendai virus.

180   Interferon alfa-2a
76543-88-9   5016
Interferon alfa-a.
alferon; alfa interferon; IFN-α; LeIF;
leukocyte interferon; lymphoblastoid
interferon; Ro-22-8181; roferon A.
Antineoplastic   agent   and
immunomodulator. Alpha interferon,
natural (injectable form); used for the
treatment of genital warts. *Hoffmann-
LaRoche Inc.*

181   Interferon alfa-2b
99210-65-8   5016
Interferon alfa-b.
intron A. Antineoplastic agent and
immunomodulator. *Schering Corp.*

182   Interferon beta
74899-71-1
Beta interferon.
fibroblast interferon. Antineoplastic agent
and immunomodulator.

183   Interferon beta-1a
145258-61-3
Interferon beta-1 human fibroblast
protein moiety.
Neoferon. Antineoplastic agent and
immunomodulator. *Biogen, Inc.*

184   Interferon beta-1b
145155-23-3   5017
17-L-Serine-2-166 interferon β1 (human
fibroblast reduced).
betaseron. Antineoplastic agent and
immunomodulator. *Berlex Labs., Inc.*

185   Interferon gamma-1a
98059-18-8   5018
Interferon gamma-a.
Antineoplastic agent; immunomodulator.
Berlex Labs., Inc.

186   Interferon gamma-1b
98059-61-1   5018
N^2-L-Methionyl-1-139-interferon-γ
(human lymphocyte protein moiety
reduced).
Actimmune. Antineoplastic agent and
immunomodulator. *Genentech, Inc.*

187   Iodothiouracil
5984-97-4

$C_4H_3IN_2OS$
5-Iodo-2-thiouracil.
Antineoplastic, used with iodine isotopes
for treatment and diagnosis.

188   Iproplatin
62928-11-4

$C_6H_{20}Cl+62N_2O_2Pt$
ab-Dichloro-cd-dihydroxy-df-
bis(isopropylamine)-platinum.
CHIP; Iproplatin (USAN); NSC-256927;
JM-9. Antineoplastic agent. *Bristol-Myers
Squibb Pharmaceutical Res. and Dev.*

189   Irinotecan
97682-44-5   5104

$C_{33}H_{38}N_4O_6$
(+)-7-Ethyl-10-hydroxycamptothecine
10-[1,4'-bipiperidine]-1'-carboxylate.
Antineoplastic   agent.   DNA

topoisomerase I inhibitor. mp = 222-223°. *Pharmacia & Upjohn, Inc.*

190   Irinotecan Hydrochloride Trihydrate
136572-09-3   5104

$C_{33}H_{39}ClN_4O_6.3H_2O$
(+)-7-Ethyl-10-hydroxycamptothecine 10-[1,4'-bipiperidine]-1'-carboxylate monohydrochloride trihydrate.
Camptosar; U-101440E. Antineoplastic agent. mp = 256.5°; $[\alpha]_D^{20}$= 67.7° (H_2O, c = 1); λ_m = 221, 254, 359, 372 nm (ε 53800, 36600, 26200, 25300, EtOH); LD_{50} (mus ip) = 177.5 mg/kg, (mus orl) = 765.3 mg/kg. *Pharmacia & Upjohn, Inc.*

191   Isotretinoin
4759-48-2   8333

$C_{20}H_{28}O_2$
3,7-Dimethyl-9-(2,6,6-trimethyl-1-cyclohexen-1-yl)-2,(E),4,6,8(Z,Z,Z)-nonatetraenoic acid.
Accutane; 13-cis-vitamin A acid; 13-cis-retinoic acid; cis-retinoic acid; neovitamin a acid; 13-RA; Ro-4-3780; retinoic acid, 9Z form; Isotretinoin; Accure; IsotrexGel; Roaccutane. mp = 174-175°; λ_m = 354 nm (ε 39800); LD_{50} (mus ip 20 day) = 904 mg/kg, (rat ip 20 day) = 901 mg/kg, (mus orl 20 day) = 3389 mg/kg, (rat orl 20 day) > 4000 mg/kg.

192   Istin
15663-27-1   2378   239-733-8

$Cl_2H_6N_2Pt$
(SP-4-2)-Diamminedichloroplatinum.
cis-diamminedichloroplatinum; cis-platinum II; cis-DDP; CACP; CPDC; DDP; Briplatin; Cismaplat; Cisplatyl; Citoplatino; Lederplatin; Neoplatin; Platamine; Platinex; Platiblastin; Platinol; Platinoxan; Platistin; Platosin; Rand; NSC-119875. Antineoplastic agent. mp = 270° (dec); soluble in H_2O (253 mg/100g), insoluble in organic solvents; LD_{50} (gpg ip) = 9.7 mg/kg. *Lederle Labs.*

193   Letrozole
112809-51-5   5474

$C_{17}H_{11}N_5$
4,4'-(1H-1,2,4-Triazol-1-ylmethylene)-dibenzonitrile.
CGS-20267. Antineoplastic agent. mp = 181-183°. *Ciba-Geigy Corp.*

194   Leucovorin
58-05-9   4254

$C_{20}H_{23}N_7O_7$
5-Formyl-5,6,7,8-tetrahydrofolate.
5-formyltetrahydrofolate; N5-formyl-5,6,7,8-tetrahydrofolate; N5-formyl-tetrahydrofolate; Folinic acid. Antineoplastic agent. mp = 240-250° (dec); λ_m = 282

nm; $[\alpha]_D^{20} = 14.26°$ (anhydrous calcium salt, c = 3.42). *Glaxo Wellcome Inc.*

LY-264618. Antineoplastic agent. *Eli Lilly & Co.*

195 Liarozole Hydrochloride
145858-50-0

$C_{17}H_{14}Cl_2N_4$
(±)-5-(m-Chloro-α-imidazol-1-yl-benzyl)benzimidazole monhydrochloride.
R-75251. Antineoplastic agent. *Janssen Pharmaceutical Inc.*

196 Lobaplatin
135558-11-1

$C_9H_{18}N_2O_3Pt$
cis-[trans-1,2-Cyclobutane-bis(methylamine)][(S)-lactato-O^1,O^1]-platinum.
D-19466. Platinum-based cytostatic drug. Antineoplastic.

197 Lometrexol
106400-81-1

$C_{21}H_{25}N_5O_6$
N-[p-[2-[(R)-2-Amino-3,4,5,6,7,8-hexahydro-4-oxopyrido[2,3-d]pyrimidin-6-yl]ethyl]benzoyl]-L-glutamic acid.

198 Lometrexol Sodium
120408-07-3

$C_{21}H_{23}Na_2N_5O_6$
N-[p-[2-[(R)-2-Amino-3,4,5,6,7,8-hexahydro-4-oxopyrido[2,3-d]pyrimidin-6-yl]ethyl]benzoyl]-L-glutamic acid disodium salt.
LY-264618 disodium. Antineoplastic agent. *Eli Lilly & Co.*

199 Lomustine
13010-47-4   5594

$C_9H_{16}ClN_3O_2$
N-(2-Chloroethyl)-N'-cyclohexyl-N-nitroso-urea.
Belustine; Cecenu; CeeNU; chloroethylcyclohexylnitrosourea; CiNu; CCNU; ICIG-1109; NSC-79037; NCI-C04740; SRI-2200. Antineoplastic agent. mp = 90°; soluble in H_2O, organic solvents; LD_{50} (mus orl) = 51 mg/kg, (mus ip) = 56 mg/kg, (mus sc) = 61 mg/kg. *Bristol-Myers Oncology.*

200 Lonidamine
50264-69-2   5598

$C_{15}H_{10}Cl_2N_2O_2$
1-(2,4-Dichlorobenzyl)-1H-imidazole-3-carboxylic acid.
Antineoplastic agent (adjunct). mp = 207°; soluble in MeOH, AcOH; LD_{50} (mus orl)= 900 mg/kg, (mus ip) = 435 mg/kg, (rat orl) = 1700 mg/kg, (rat ip) = 525 mg/kg.

201 Losoxantrone
88303-60-0

$C_{22}H_{27}N_5O_4$
7-Hydroxy-2-[2-[(2-hydroxyethyl)amino]-ethyl]-5-[[2-[(2-hydroxyethyl)amino]-ethyl]amino]anthra[1,9-cd]-pyrazol-6(2H)-one.
biantrazole. Antineoplastic agent. *DuPont Merck Pharmaceutical Co.*

202 Losoxantrone Hydrochloride
88303-61-1

$C_{22}H_{29}Cl_2N_5O_4 \cdot 0.5H_2O$
7-Hydroxy-2-[2-[(2-hydroxyethyl)amino]-ethyl]-5-[[2-[(2-hydroxyethyl)amino]-ethyl]amino]anthra[1,9-cd]pyrazol-6(2H)-one dihydrochloride hemihydrate. DUP-941; NSC-357885. Antineoplastic agent. *DuPont Merck Pharmaceutical Co.*

203 Lurtotecan
149882-10-0

$C_{28}H_{30}N_4O_6$
(8S)-8-Ethyl-2,3-dihydro-8-hydroxy-15-[(4-methyl-1-piperazinyl)methyl]-11H-p-dioxino[2,3-g]pyrano[3',4':6,7]-indolizino[1,2-b]quinoline-9,12(8H,14H)-dione.
Antineoplastic agent. DNA topo-isomerase I inhibitor. *Glaxo Wellcome Inc.*

204 Lurtotecan Dihydrochloride
155773-58-3

$C_{28}H_{32}Cl_2N_4O_6$
(8S)-8-Ethyl-2,3-dihydro-8-hydroxy-15-[(4-methyl-1-piperazinyl)methyl]-11H-p-dioxino[2,3-g]pyrano[3',4':6,7]-indolizino[1,2-b]quinoline-9,12(8H,14H)-dione.
GI-147211C.

205 Mafosfamide
88859-04-5

$C_9H_{19}Cl_2N_2O_5PS_2$
(±)-2-[[2-[Bis(2-chloroethyl)amino]tetra-hydro-2H-1,3,2-oxazaphosphorin-4-yl]-thio]ethanesulfonic acid P-cis-oxide.
Antineoplastic; immunosuppressant. A cyclophosphamide deriviative.

206   Mannomustine Hydrochloride
551-74-6

$$ClH_2CH_2CHNH_2C \overset{H\ \ H\ OHOH}{\underset{OHOH\ H\ \ H}{\rule{2.5cm}{0.4pt}}} CH_2NHCH_2CH_2Cl$$
H–Cl

$C_{10}H_{24}Cl_4N_2O_4$
1,6-bis[(2-Chloroethyl)amino]-1,6-dideoxy-D-mannitol hydrochloride.
BCM; Degranol; Degranol chinoin; Dimesylmannitol; Mannitol mustard dihydrochloride; NSC-9698; Mannitol nitrogen mustard; Mannogranol; Mannomustine dihydrochloride. Antineoplastic agent.

207   Mannosulfan
7518-35-6

$$H_3CO_2SO \underset{HO}{\overset{OSO_2CH_3}{\rule{1.8cm}{0.4pt}}} \begin{array}{l} OH \\ OSO_2CH_3 \\ OSO_2CH_3 \end{array}$$

$C_{10}H_{22}O_{14}S_4$
D-Mannitol 1,2,5,6-tetramethanesulfonate.
R-52. Antineoplastic.

208   Masoprocol
27686-84-6   6786

meso-4,4'-(2,3-Dimethyltetramethylene)-dipyrocatachol.
CHX-100; meso-NDGA; Actinex. Antineoplastic agent. an antioxidant for fats and oils in foods. mp = 185-186°; λ_m = 283, 218 nm (ε 6660, 13400 MeOH); poorly soluble in H_2O, more soluble in

EtOH, insoluble in non-polar organic solvents. *Schwarz Pharma Kremers Urban Co.*

209   Matulane
366-70-1   7938   206-678-6

$C_{12}H_{20}ClN_3O$
N-(1-Methylethyl)-4-[(2-methylhydrazino)methyl]benzamide monohydrochloride.
procarbazine hydrochloride; ibenzmethyzine hydrochloride; Matulane; MBH; MIH hydrochloride; Nathulane; Natulan; NSC-77213; Natunalar; NCI-C01810; Procarbazin; PCB hydrochloride; Ro-4-6467/1. Antineoplastic agent. mp = 223-226°; LD_{50} (rat orl) = 785 mg/kg. *Hoffmann-LaRoche Inc.*

210   Maytansine
35846-53-8   5800

$C_{34}H_{46}ClN_3O_{10}$
N-Acetyl-N-methyl alanine 6-ester with 11-chloro-6,21-dihydroxy-12,20-dimethoxy-2,5,9,16-tetramethyl-4,24-dioxa-9,22-diazatetracyclo-[19.3.1.1(10,24).0(3,5)]hexacosa-10,12,14[26]16,18-pentaene-8,23-dione.
Maitansine; Maysanine; Maytansin; Maytansine; MTS; NSC-153858. Antineoplastic agent. mp= 171-172°; $[\alpha]_D^{26}$= -145° (CHCl$_3$ c = 0.055); λ_m = 233, 254, 282, 290 nm (ε 29800, 27200, 5690, 5520,

EtOH); LD$_{50}$ (rat sc) = 0.48 mg/kg. *Bristol-Myers Squibb Pharmaceutical.*

211 Mechlorethamine
51-75-2   5815   200-120-5

C$_5$H$_{11}$Cl$_2$N
N,N-Bis(2-chloroethyl)methylamine.
MBA; Nitrogen Mustard; Mechloro-ethamine; HN-2; Mustine Note; Dichloren; Caryolysine. Antineoplastic agent. mp = -60°; bp$_{18}$ = 87°; d$_4^{25}$= 1.118; slightly soluble in H$_2$O, soluble in organic solvents; LD$_{50}$ (rat iv) = 1.1 mg/kg (hydrochloride). *Merck & Co., Inc.*

212 Mechlorethamine Hydrochloride
55-86-7   5815

C$_5$H$_{12}$Cl$_3$N
N,N-Bis(2-chloroethyl)methylamine monohydrochloride.
Azotoyperite; C-6866; Caryolysine hydrochloride; Chloramin hydrochloride; Chlorethamine; Chlorethazine; Chlor-methine hydrochloride; Chlormethinum; Dema; Dichloren hydrochloride; Dichloromethyldiethylamine hydro-chloride; Dimitan; Embechine; Embichin hydrochloride; NSC-762; Embikhine; Erasol hydrochloride; Erasol-Ido; HN2 hydrochloride; Mechlorethamine hydro-chloride; Mitoxine; Mustargen hydro-chloride; Mustine hydrochloride; MBA hydrochloride; N-Lost; Nitol; Nitol takeda; Nitrogen mustard hydrochloride;

Nitrogranulogen hydrochloride; NCI-C56382; NM; SK-101. Antineoplastic agent. *Merck & Co., Inc.*

213 Medorubicin
64314-52-9

C$_{26}$H$_{27}$NO$_{10}$
(7S-cis)-7-[(3-Amino-2,3,6-trideoxy-α-L-lyxo-hexopyranosyl)oxy]-7,8,9,10-tetrahydro-6,9,11-trihydroxy-9-(hydroxyacetyl)-5,12-naphthacenedione.
Medorubicin; 4-DMA; 4-demethoxy-adriamycin. Antineoplastic agent.

214 Medorubicin Hydrochloride
64363-63-9

C$_{26}$H$_{28}$ClNO$_{10}$
(7S-cis)-7-[(3-Amino-2,3,6-trideoxy-α-L-lyxo-hexopyranosyl)oxy]-7,8,9,10-tetrahydro-6,9,11-trihydroxy-9-(hydroxyacetyl)-5,12-naphthacenedione hydrochloride.
medorubicin hydrochloride; 4-DMA HCl; 4-demethoxyadriamycin HCl; NSC-256438. Antineoplastic agent.

215   Menogaril
71628-96-1   5881

$C_{28}H_{31}NO_{10}$
4-(Dimethylamino)-3,4,5,6,11,12,13,14-octahydro-3,5,8,10,13-pentahydroxy-11-methoxy-6,13-dimethyl 2,6-epoxy-2H-naphthaceno[1,2-b]oxocin-9,16-dione.
U-52047; 7(R)-O-Methylnogarol; 7-O-Methylnogarol; 7-OMEN; NSC-269148.
Antineoplastic agent. mp = 247-249° (dec), 250-254° (dec); $[\alpha]_D^{20}$= 857° (CHCl$_3$ c = 0.112), 867° (CHCl$_3$ c = 0.045); 958° (CHCl$_3$ c = 0.163); λ_m = 235, 251, 257, 290, 479 (ϵ 41200, 25500, 24150, 10500, 15530 EtOH). *Upjohn Ltd.*

216   Mequinol
150-76-5   205-769-8

$C_7H_8O_2$
4-Methoxyphenol.
Antioxidant. Studied for its utility in treatment of malignant melanomas.

217   6-Mercaptopurine
50-44-2   5919   200-037-4

$C_5H_4N_4S$
1,7-Dihydro-6H-purine-6-thione.
mercaptopurine; purine-6-thiol; thio-hypoxanthine; Ismipur; Leukeran; Leukerin; Leupurin; Mercaleukim; Mercaleukin; Mercapurin; Mern; Puri-Nethol; Purimethol; Purinethiol; U-4748; 3H-purine-6-thiol; 6 MP; 6-purinethiol; 6-thioxopurine; 7-mercapto-1,3,4,6-tetrazaindene; 6-purinethiol hydrate; NSC-755. Antineoplastic, immunosuppressant. Dec 313-314°; λ_m = 230, 312 nm (ϵ 14000, 19600 0.1N NaOH); insoluble in H$_2$O, organic solvents; slightly soluble in EtOH; LD$_{50}$ (mus ip) = 157 mg/kg.

218   Metamelfalan
1088-80-8

$C_{13}H_{18}Cl_2N_2O_2$
3-[m-[Bis(2-chloroethyl)amino]phenyl]-L-alanine.
L-m-Sarcolysin; NSC-67781. Antineoplastic agent.

219   Metesind
138384-68-6

$C_{23}H_{24}N_4O_3S$
4-[[α-[(2-Aminobenz[c,d]indol-6-yl)-methylamino]-p-tolyl]sulfonyl]-morpholine.
Antineoplastic agent. Thymidylate synthase inhibitor. *Agouron Pharmaceuticals, Inc.*

220 Metesind Glucuronate
157182-23-5

$C_{29}H_{34}N_4O_{10}S$
4-[[α-[(2-Aminobenz[c,d]indol-6-yl)-methylamino]-p-tolyl]sulfonyl]-morpholine mono-D-glucuronate.
AG-331. Antineoplastic agent. Thymidylate synthase inhibitor. *Agouron Pharmaceuticals, Inc.*

221 Methotrexate
59-05-2   6065   200-413-8

$C_{20}H_{22}N_8O_5$
L-(+)-N-[[(2,4-Diamino-6-pteridinyl)-methyl]methylamino]benzoyl]glutamic acid.
Amethopterin; CL-14377; EMT-25299; HDMTX; Metatrexan; Methopterin; NSC-740; Methylaminopterin; MTX; NCI-C04671; R-9985; CL-14377. Antineoplastic agent. mp = 185-204°; λ_m = 244, 307 nm (0.1N HCl); LD_{50} (rat orl) = 135 mg/kg. *Bristol-Myers Oncology.*

222 Methylthiouracil
56-04-2   6210

$C_5H_6N_2OS$
2,3-Dihydro-6-methyl-2-thioxo-4(1H)-pyrimidinone.

NSC-193526; Antibason; Basecil; Basethyrin; Methiacil; Methicil; Methiocil; Methylthiouracil; Muracil; Muracin; MTU; Orcanon; Prostrumyl; Strumacil; Thimecil; Thiomecil; Thiomidil; Thioryl; NSC-9378; Thiothymin; Thiothyron; Thiuryl; Thyreonorm; Thyreostat; Thyreostat I; Thyril; Tiomeracil; Tiorale M; Tiotiron; USAF EK-6454; 4-methyluracil; 6-methyl-2-thiouracil. Antineoplastic agent. Thyroid inhibitor. mp = 326-331° (dec); slightly soluble in H_2O, EtOH, Et_2O; insoluble in other organic solvents; MLD (rbt orl) = 2500 mg/kg.

223 Metoprine
7761-45-7

$C_{11}H_{10}Cl_2N_4$
5-(3,4-Dichlorophenyl)-6-methyl-2,4-pyrimidinediamine.
NSC-19494; BW-197U; BW-50197; DDMP; Methodichlorophen; SK-5265; U-197; NSC-7364. Antineoplastic agent.

224 Meturedepa
1661-29-6   6245

$C_{11}H_{22}N_3O_3P$
Ethyl [bis(2,2-dimethyl-1-aziridinyl)-phosphinyl]carbamate.
AB-132; Turloc; NSC-51325. Antineoplastic agent. mp = 119-121°.

225   Miltefosine
58066-85-6   6285

$C_{21}H_{46}NO_4P$
Choline hydroxide hexadecyl hydrogen phosphate inner salt.
hexadecylphosphorylcholine; D-18506; HPC; Miltex. Antineoplastic. mp = 232-234° (dec); LD_{50} (rat orl) = 246 mg/kg.

226   Miproxifene
129612-87-9

$C_{29}H_{35}NO_2$
(Z)-α-[p-[2-(Dimethylamino)ethoxy]-phenyl]-α'-ethyl-4'-isopropyl-4-stilbenol. TAT-59 [as phosphate]. Antineoplastic.

227   Mithramycin
18378-89-7   7696   232-455-8

$C_{22}H_{38}O_5$
[2S-[2α,3β(1R*,3R*,4S*)]]-6-[[2,6-Dideoxy-3-O-(2,6-dideoxy-β-D-arabino-hexopyranosyl)-β-D-arabino-hexopyranosyl]oxy]-2-[(O-2,6-dideoxy-3-C-methyl-β-D-ribo-hexopyranosyl-(1→4)-O-2,6-dideoxy-α-D-lyxo-hexopyranosyl-(1→3)-2,6-dideoxy-β-D-arabino-hexopyranosyl)oxy]-3-(3,4-dihydroxy-1-methoxy-2-oxopentyl)-3,4-dihydro-8,9-dihydroxy-7-methyl-1(2H)-anthracenone.
A-2371; Antibiotic LA-7017; Aurelic acid; Aureolic acid; Mithracin; Mithramycin A; Mitramycin; PA-144; NSC-24559; plicamycin. Antineoplastic agent. mp = 180-183°; $[α]_D^{20}$= 51° (c = 0.4 EtOH); soluble in H_2O, polar organic solvents; less soluble in Et_2O, C_6H_6; LD_{50} (rat iv) = 1.74 mg/kg. *Bayer Corp., Pharmaceutical Div.*

228   Mitindomide
10403-51-7

$C_{14}H_{12}N_2O_4$
(3aα,3bβ,4α,4aβ,7aβ,8α,8aβ,8bα)-3a,3b,4,4a,7a,8,8a,8b-Octahydro-4,8-ethenopyrrolo[3',4':3,4]cyclobut[1,2-f]-isoindole-1,3,5,7(2H,6H)tetrone. Benzenebismaleimide adduct; Mitindomide; NSC-284356. Antineoplastic agent. *National Cancer Inst.*

229   Mitobronitol
488-41-5   6298

$C_6H_{12}Br_2O_4$
1,6-Dibromo-1,6-dideoxy-D-mannitol. D-dibromomannitol; Dibromannit; Dibromannitol; Dibromomannitol; Mielobromol; NSC-94100; Mitobronitol; Myelobromol; NCI-C04762; R-54; 1,6-dibromo-D-mannitol; 1,6-dibromo-1,6-dideoxy-D-mannitol; 1,6-Dibromo-mannitol. Antineoplastic agent. mp = 176-178°.

230 Mitocarcin
11056-14-7
Antineoplastic agent. Antibiotic derived from *Streptomyces* species.

231 Mitocromin
11043-98-4
B-35251; NSC-77471. Antineoplastic agent. Antibiotic derived from *Streptomyces viridochromogenes* species.

232 Mitogillin
1403-99-2
Antineoplastic agent. Antibiotic produced by *Aspergillus restrictus*.

233 Mitoguazone
459-86-9   6299

$C_5H_{12}N_8$
1,1'-[(Methylethanediylidene)dinitrilo]di-guanidine.
Antineoplastic agent. mp = 225° (dec); λ_m = 283 nm (ε 38400 pH 1), 325 nm (ε 33500 pH 11).

234 Mitolactol
10318-26-0   6300

$C_6H_{12}Br_2O_4$
1,6-Dibromo-1,6-dideoxy-D-galactitol.
Dibromdulcit; Dibromdulcitol; Dibromo-dulcitol; Dibromogalactitol; DBD; Elo-

bromol; NSC-104800; NCI-C04795. Antineoplastic agent. mp = 187-188°; LD_{50} (rat orl) = 1400 mg/kg, (rat ip) = 470 mg/kg.

235 Mitomalcin
11043-99-5
NSC-113233. Antineoplastic agent. Antibiotic produced by *Streptomyces malayensis*. *Pfizer International*.

236 Mitomycin
50-07-7

$C_{15}H_{18}N_4O_5$
(1aS,8S,8aR,8bS)-6-Amino-1,1a,2,8,8a,8b-hexahydro-8-(hydroxymethyl)-8a-methoxy-5-methylazirino[2',3':3,4]pyrrolo[1,2-a]-indole-4,7-dione carbamate (ester).
Mutamycin; Mitomycin C; MMC; Ametycine; NSC-26980. Antineoplastic agent. *Bristol-Myers Oncology*.

237 Mitonafide
54824-17-8

$C_{16}H_{15}N_3O_4$
N-[2-(Dimethylamino)ethyl]-3-nitronaphthalimide.
Non-cationic tricyclic aromatic carboxamide cytotoxic agent. Antineoplastic Agent.

238   Mitopodozide
1508-45-8   7703

$C_{24}H_{30}N_2O_8$
Podophyllic acid 2-ethylhydrazide.
SPI-77;   NSC-72274.   Antineoplastic
agent. $[\alpha]_D$= -154° (CHCl$_3$ c = 0.5).

239   Mitoquidone
91753-07-0

$C_{20}H_{13}NO_2$
5,14-Dihydrobenz[5,6]isoindolo[2,1-b]-
isoquinoline-8,13-dione.
GR-30921.   A   pentacyclic
pyrroloquinone. Antineoplastic.

240   Mitosper
11056-15-8
NSC-117032. Antineoplastic agent. *State
of Michigan Department of Public
Health.*

241   Mitotane
53-19-0   6302   200-166-6

$C_{14}H_{10}Cl_4$
1,1-Dichloro-2-(o-chlorophenyl)-2-(p-
chlorophenyl)ethane.
Lysodren;   o,p'-DDE;   NSC-38721.

Antineoplastic agent. mp = 76-78°;
soluble in EtOH, isooctane, CCl$_4$. *Bristol-
Myers Oncology.*

242   Mitoxana
3778-73-2   4937   223-237-3

$C_7H_{15}Cl_2N_2O_2P$
3-(2-Chloroethyl)-2-[(2-chloroethyl)-
amino]tetrahydro-2H-1,3,2-oxaza-
phosphorine 2-oxide.
Isophosphamide;   Ifex;   Iphosphamid;
Isoendoxan; Cyfos; Holoxan; Mitoxana;
Naxamide; A-4942; Asta-Z-4942; NSC-
109724;   Holoxan   1000;   Ifosfamid;
Iphosphamid; Isofosfamide; MJF-9325; Z-
4942. Antineoplastic agent. mp = 39-41°;
LD$_{50}$ (rat ip) = 150 mg/kg, 160 mg/kg.
Bristol-Myers Oncology.

243   Mitoxantrone
65271-80-9   6303

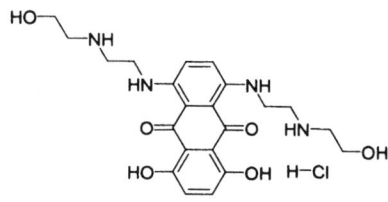

$C_{22}H_{28}N_4O_6$
1,4-Dihydroxy-5,8-bis[[2-[(2-hydroxy-
ethyl)amino]ethyl]amino]-9,10-
anthracenedione.
Dihydroxyanthraquinone;   DHAQ;
Mitoxantrone [as free base]; NSC-
279836. Antineoplastic agent. mp = 160-
162°; λ_m = 244, 279, 525, 620, 660 nm
(log ε 4.64, 4.31, 3.70, 4.37, 4.38 EtOH);
sparingly   soluble   in   H$_2$O,   EtOH;
insoluble in organic solvents.

244 Mitoxantrone Dihydrochloride
70476-82-3   6303

$C_{22}H_{30}Cl_2N_4O_6$
1,4-Dihydroxy-5,8-bis[[2-[(2-hydroxy-ethyl)amino]ethyl]amino]-9,10-anthracenedione dihydrochloride.
DHAQ; CL232315; NSC-279836; Novantrone; Immunex; CL-232315. Antineoplastic agent. mp = 203-205°; λ_m = 241, 273, 608, 658 nm (ε 41000, 12000, 19200, 20900 H_2O); sparingly soluble in H_2O, MeOH; insoluble in organic solvents.

245 Mitozolomide
85622-95-3   287-943-3

$C_7H_7ClN_6O_2$
3-(2-Chloroethyl)-3,4-dihydro-4-oxoimidazo[5,1-d]-as-tetrazine-8-carboxamide.
M&B-39565; NSC-353451. Antitumor bicyclic imidazotetrazine; a chloroethylating agent. Antineoplastic.

246 Mivobulin Isethionate
126268-81-3

$C_{17}H_{19}N_5O_2 \cdot C_2H_6O_4S$
Ethyl (S)-5-amino-1,2-dihydro-2-methyl-3-phenylpyrido[3,4-b]pyrazine-7-carbamate

mono(2-hydroxyethanesulfonate).
BW-B1090U; Mivacron; CI-980. Antineoplastic agent. Microtubule inhibitor. *Parke-Davis*.

247 Mofarotene
125533-88-2

$C_{29}H_{39}NO_2$
4-[2-[p-[(E)-2-(5,6,7,8-Tetrahydro-5,5,8,8-tetramethyl-2-naphthyl)-propenyl]phenoxy]ethyl]morpholine.
Ro-40-8757. Retinoid analog. Antineoplastic.

248 Momordicine
$C_9H_{14}N_4O_4$
N-(Ethoxycarbonyl)-3-(4-morpholinyl)-sydnone imine.
morsydomine; SIN-10; Corvaton; Corvasal; Molsidolat; Morial; Motazomin; Molsidain; Molsidaine. Antianginal.

249 Mopidamol
13665-88-8   6344

$C_{19}H_{31}N_7O_4$
2,2',2,2'''-[(4-Piperidinopyrimido[5,4-d]-pyrimidine-2,6-diyl)dintrilo]tetraethanol.
RA-233; Rapenton. Antineoplastic agent. Platelet aggregation inhibitor with antimetastatic properties. mp = 157-158°.

250   Moss Starch
1402-10-4   5503   215-755-3

$C_{18}H_{32}O_{15}$
Lichenin.
Antineoplastic agent. Soluble in H_2O;
$[\alpha]_D = 18.4°$.

251   Mustargen®
55-86-7   5815

$C_5H_{12}Cl_3N$
N,N-Bis(2-chloroethyl)methylamine
monohydrochloride.
Azotoyperite; C 6866; Caryolysine
hydrochloride; Chloramin hydrochloride;
Chlorethamine; Chlorethazine;
Chlormethine hydrochloride;
Chlormethinum; Dema; Dichloren
hydrochloride;
Dichloromethyldiethylamine
hydrochloride; Dimitan; Embechine;
Embichin hydrochloride; NSC-762;
Embikhine; Erasol hydrochloride; Erasol-
Ido; HN2 hydrochloride;
Mechlorethamine hydrochloride;
Mitoxine; Mustargen hydrochloride;
Mustine hydrochloride; MBA
hydrochloride; N-Lost; Nitol; Nitol
takeda; Nitrogen mustard hydrochloride;
Nitrogranulogen hydrochloride; NCI-
C56382; NM; SK 101. Antineoplastic
agent. *Merck & Co., Inc.*

252   Mustine
55-86-7   5815

$C_5H_{12}Cl_3N$
N,N-Bis(2-chloroethyl)methylamine
monohydrochloride.
Azotoyperite; C 6866; Caryolysine
hydrochloride; Chloramin hydrochloride;
Chlorethamine; Chlorethazine;
Chlormethine hydrochloride;
Chlormethinum; Dema; Dichloren
hydrochloride; Dichloromethyldiethylamine hydrochloride; Dimitan;
Embechine; Embichin hydrochloride;
NSC-762; Embikhine; Erasol
hydrochloride; Erasol-Ido; HN2
hydrochloride; Mechlorethamine
hydrochloride; Mitoxine; Mustargen
hydrochloride; Mustine hydrochloride;
MBA hydrochloride; N-Lost; Nitol; Nitol
takeda; Nitrogen mustard hydrochloride;
Nitrogranulogen hydrochloride; NCI-
C56382; NM; SK 101. Antineoplastic
agent. *Merck & Co., Inc.*

253   Mutamycin
50-07-7   6301   200-008-6

$C_{15}H_{18}N_4O_5$
(1aS,8S,8aR,8bS)-6-Amino-
1,2a,2,8,8a,8b-hexahydro-8-
(hydroxymethyl)-8A-methoxy-5-
methylazirino[2',3':3,4]pyrrolo[1,2-
a]indole-4,7-dione carbamate (ester).
Mitomycin; Mitomycin C; MMC;
Ametycine; NSC-26980. Antineoplastic
agent. mp > 360°; soluble in H_2O,
organic solvents; λ_m = 216, 360, 560 nm
($E_{1\ cm}^{1\%}$ 742, 742, 0.06 MeOH); LD_{50} (mus
iv) = 5 mg/kg. *Bristol-Myers Oncology.*

254   Mycophenolic Acid
24280-93-1   6408

$C_{17}H_{20}O_6$
(E)-6-(1,3-Dihydro-4-hydroxy-6-methoxy-7-methyl-3-oxo-5-isobenzofuranyl)-4-methyl-4-hexenoic acid.
Melbex; Lilly 68618; MPA; NSC-129185. Antineoplastic agent. mp = 141°; insoluble in H_2O, soluble in organic solvents; LD_{50} (mus orl) = 2500 mg/kg, (mus iv) = 550 mg/kg, (rat orl) = 700 mg/kg, (rat iv) = 450 mg/kg. *Eli Lilly & Co.*

255   Myleran
55-98-1   1529   200-250-2

$C_6H_{14}O_6S_2$
1,4-Butanediol dimethanesulfonate.
AN-33501; Busulfan; Busulphan; Buzulfan; Citosulfan; CB-2041; GT-2041; GT-41; Leucosulfan; Mablin; Mielevcin; Mielosan; Mielucin; Milecitan; Mileran; Misulban; NSC-750; Mitostan; Myeloleukon; Myelosan; Mylecytan; Myleran Tablets; NCI-C01592; Sulphabutin; X-149; 1,4-Bis(methanesulfonyloxy)butane; 2041 C.B. Antineoplastic agent. A proprietary preparation containing cyclopentolate hydrochloride; an antimuscarinic agent; eye drops. mp = 114-118°; insoluble in H_2O, soluble in organic solvents; LD_{50} (mus iv) = 1.8 mg/kg. *Glaxo Wellcome Inc.*

256   Mylosar
320-67-2   923

$C_8H_{12}N_4O_5$
4-Amino-1-β-D-ribofuranosyl-1,3,5-triazin-2(1H)-one.
5-azacytidine; ladakamycin; U-18496; NSC-102816. Antineoplastic agent. mp = 228-230°; $[\alpha]_D^{25}$ = 39° (H_2O, c = 1); λ_m = 241 nm (ε 8767 H_2O), 249 nm (ε 3077 0.01N HCl), 223 nm (ε 24200 0.01N KOH); LD_{50} (mus ip) = 115.9 mg/kg, (mus orl) = 572.3 mg/kg. *Pharmacia & Upjohn, Inc.*

257   Natulan
366-70-1   7938   206-678-6

$C_{12}H_{20}ClN_3O$
N-(1-Methylethyl)-4-[(2-methylhydrazino) methyl]-benzamide monohydrochloride.
procarbazine hydrochloride; Ibenzmethyzine hydrochloride; Matulane; MBH; MIH hydrochloride; Nathulane; Natulan; NSC-77213; Natunalar; NCI-C01810; Procarbazin; PCB hydrochloride; Ro-4-6467/1. Antineoplastic agent. mp = 223-226°; LD_{50} (rat orl) = 785 mg/kg. *Hoffmann-LaRoche Inc.*

258   Nedaplatin
95734-82-0

$C_2H_8N_2O_3Pt$
cis-Diammine(glycolato-O^1,O^2)platinum.
Antineoplastic agent.

259   Nemorubicin
108852-90-0

$C_{32}H_{37}NO_{13}$
(1S,3S)-3-Glycoloyl-1,2,3,4,6,11-
hexahydro-3,5,12-trihydroxy-10-
methoxy-6,11-dioxo-1-naphthacenyl
2,3,6-trideoxy-3-[(S)-2-
methoxymorpholino]-α-L-lyxo-
hexopyranoside.
Antineoplastic agent.

260   Neosar
50-18-0   2816   200-015-4

$C_7H_{15}Cl_2N_2O_2P$
(Bis(chloro-2-ethyl)amino)-2-tetrahydro-
3,4,5,6-oxazaphosphorine-1,3,2-oxide-2
hydrate.
ASTA-B-518;   Clafen;   Claphene;
Cyclophosphamid;   Cyclophosphamide;
Cyclophosphamidum;   Cyclophosphan;
Cyclophosphane;   Cyclostin;   Cytophos-
phan; Cytoxan; NSC-26271; CB-4564;
CP; CPA; CTX; CY; Endoxan; Endoxan R;

Endoxan-Asta;   Endoxana;   Endoxanal;
Endoxane; Enduxan; Genoxal; Hexadrin;
Mitoxan; Neosar; NCI-C04900; Procytox;
Semdoxan; Sendoxan; Senduxan; SK-
20501; Zyklophosphamid. Antineoplastic
agent. mp = 41-45°; soluble in H_2O (40
g/l), less soluble in oganic solvents; LD_{50}
(rat orl) = 94 mg/kg. *Pharmacia &*
Upjohn, Inc.

261   Nigrin
3930-19-6   8986   223-501-8

$C_{25}H_{22}N_4O_8$
5-Amino-6-(7-amino-5,8-dihydro-6-
methoxy-5,8-dioxo-2-quinolyl)-4-
(2-hydroxy-3,4-dimethoxyphenyl)-3-
methylpicolinic acid.
streptonigrin;   Abbott   Crystalline
antibiotic; AO50165L302; NSC-45383;
Bruneomycin; Nigrin; Rufochrommycin;
Rufocromomycin; Streptonigran; STP;
5278 R.P. Antineoplastic agent. Antitumor antibiotic from *Streptomyces
flocculus.* mp= 262-263° (dec); λ_m = 248,
375-380 nm (ε 38400, 17400, MeOH);
slightly soluble in H_2O, alcohols; more
soluble in dioxane, C_5H_5N, DMF. *Pfizer
Inc.*

262   Nimustine
42471-28-3   6645

$C_9H_{13}ClN_6O_2$
3-[(-4-Amino-2-methyl-5-pyrimidinyl)-
methyl]-1-(2-chloroethyl)-1-nitrosourea.

9-methylfolic acid; Bremfol. Antineoplastic agent. mp = 125° (dec).

263 Nimustine Hydrochloride
55661-38-6   6645

$C_9H_{14}Cl_2N_6O_2$
3-[(-4-Amino-2-methyl-5-pyrimidinyl)-methyl]-1-(2-chloroethyl)-1-nitrosourea hydrochloride.
ACNU;   CS-439   HCl;   Nidran hydrochloride; Nimustine hydrochloride; NSC-245382. Antineoplastic agent. λ_m = 245 nm ($E_{1\ cm}^{1\%}$ = 480-510 0.04N HCl); soluble in EtOH, less soluble in other organic solvents; LD_{50} (mus iv) = 62 mg/kg, (rat iv) = 46 mg/kg.

264 Nitracrine Hydrochloride
6514-85-8   6661

$C_{18}H_{22}Cl_2N_4O_2$
9-[[3-(Dimethylamino)propyl]amino]-1-nitroacridine dihydrochloride.
C-283;   Ledacrine;   Nitracrine dihydrochloride;   NSC-247561. Antineoplastic agent. mp = 134-135°; insoluble in H_2O, soluble in organic solvents.

265 Nocodazole
31430-18-9

$C_{14}H_{11}N_3O_3S$
[[5-(2-Thienylcarbonyl)-1H-benzimidazol-2-yl]]carbamic acid methyl ester.
Oncodazole;   R-17934; NSC-238159. Antineoplastic   agent.   *Janssen Pharmaceutical, Belgium*.

266 Nogalamycin
1404-15-5   6767

$C_{39}H_{49}NO_{16}$
(2α,3β,4α,5β,6α,11β,13α,14α)-(+)-11-[[(6-Deoxy-3-C-methyl-2,3,4-tri-O-methyl-α-L-mannopyranosyl)oxy]-4-(dimethylamino)-3,4,5,6,9,11,12,13,14,16-decahydro-3,5,8,10,13-penta-hydroxy-6,13-dimethyl-9,16-dioxo-2,6-epoxy-2H-naphthaceno[1,2-b]oxocin-14-carboxylic acid methyl ester.
Antibiotic 205t3; Nogalamycin (8CI); U-15167; NSC-70845. Antitumor antibiotic from   *Streptomyces   nogalater   var. nogalater*. mp = 195-196° (dec); $[\alpha]_D^{25}$ = 425° ($CHCl_3$ c = 0.11); λ_m = 236, 258, 292 nm (ε 52360, 24755, 9890 EtOH); insoluble in H_2O, alcohols, soluble in organic solvents; LD_{50} (mus iv) = 11.75 mg/kg, (mus ip) = 4.79 mg/kg. *Rybar Labs. Ltd*.

267   Noltam
54965-24-1   9216

$C_{32}H_{37}NO_8$
(Z)-2-[p-(1,2-Diphenyl-1-butenyl)-
phenoxy]-N,N-dimethylamine citrate.
tamoxifen citrate; ICI-46474 citrate;
Kessar; Nolvadex; Nourytam; Tamofen;
Tamozasta, Zemide; TMX; NSC-180973.
Antineoplastic agent. Antiestrogen, used
in palliative treatment of breast cancer.
mp = 140-142°; slightly soluble in H_2O;
more soluble in EtOH, MeOH, Me_2CO;
LD_{50} (mus ip) = 200 mg/kg, (mus iv) =
62.5 mg/kg, (mus orl) = 3000-6000
mg/kg, (rat ip) = 600 mg/kg), (rat iv) =
62.5 mg/kg, (rat orl) = 1200-2500 mg/kg.
ICI.

268   Nolvadex
54965-24-1   9216

$C_{32}H_{37}NO_8$
(Z)-2-[p-(1,2-Diphenyl-1-butenyl)-
phenoxy]-N,N-dimethylamine citrate.

Tamoxifen citrate; ICI-46474 citrate;
Kessar; Noltam; Nourytam; Tamofen;
Tamozasta, Zemide; TMX; NSC-180973.
Antineoplastic agent. Antiestrogen, used
in palliative treatment of breast cancer.
mp = 140-142°. *ICI.*

269   Novantrone
70476-82-3   6303

$C_{22}H_{28}N_4O_6$
Mitoxantrone hydrochloride.
Dihydroxyanthraquinone;   DHAQ;
Mitoxantrone [as free base]; NSC-
279836. Antineoplastic agent. mp = 203-
205°; λ_m = 241, 273, 608, 658 nm (ε
41000, 12000, 19200, 20900 H_2O);
sparingly soluble in H_2O, MeOH;
insoluble in organic solvents. *Immunex
Corp.*

270   Oltipraz
64224-21-1   264-736-6

$C_8H_6N_2S_3$
4-Methyl-5-(pyrazinyl)-3H-1,2-dithiole-
3-thione.
RP-35972.   Anticarcinogen.   An
antischistosomal   drug   with
chemoprotective properties.

271 Oncovin
2068-78-2 10124 200-318-1

$C_{46}H_{56}N_4O_{10}.H_2SO_4$
22-Oxo-vincaleukoblastine sulfate (1:1) (salt).
Kyocristine; Leurocristine sulfate; Lilly 37231; LCR; Oncovin; Onkovin; Vincristine sulfate; Vincrisul; VCR sulfate; 37231; NSC-67574. Antineoplastic agent. *Eli Lilly & Co.*

272 Ormaplatin
62816-98-2

$C_6H_{14}Cl_4N_2Pt$
(±)-trans-Tetrachloro(1,2-cyclohexane-diamine)platinum.
U-77233; tetraplatin; NSC-363812. Antineoplastic agent. *Pharmacia & Upjohn, Inc.*

273 Oxaliplatin
61825-94-3 7044

$C_8H_{12}N_2O_4Pt$
[(1R,2R)-1,2-Cyclohexanediamine-N,N'][oxolato(2-)-O,O']platinum.
(1R-trans)-(9CI)-1,2-cyclohexanediamine

platinum complex; trans-l-diaminocyclohexane oxalatoplatinum; oxaliplatin; dacplat; exloxatin; NSC-266046. Antineoplastic agent. Soluble in H_2O (7.9 mg/ml).

274 Oxisuran
27302-90-5

$C_8H_9NO_2S$
(Methylsulfinyl)methyl-2-pyridiyl ketone. Ismisupren; Ketone, (methylsulfinyl)-methyl 2-pyridyl; NSC-356716; 2-[(methylsulfinyl)acetyl]pyridine; W 6495. Antineoplastic agent. *Parke-Davis.*

275 Paclitaxel
33069-62-4 7117

$C_{47}H_{51}NO_{14}$
[2aR-[2aα,4β,4aβ,6β,9α-(R*,βS*),11α,12α,12aα,12bα]]-β-(Benzoylamino)-α-hydroxybenzenepropanoic acid 6,12b-bis(acetyloxy)-12-(benzoyloxy)-2a,3,4,4a,5,6,9,10,11,12,12a,12b-dodecahydro-4,11-dihydroxy-4a,8,13,13-tetramethyl-5-oxo-7,11-methano-1H-cyclodeca[3,4]benz[1,2-b]oxet-9-yl ester.
Taxol®; NSC-125973. Antineoplastic agent. Microtubule inhibitor; used in treatment of ovarian cancer. mp = 213-216° (dec); $[\alpha]_D^{20}$ = -49° (MeOH); λ_m = 227, 273 nm (ε 29800 1700 MeOH). *Bristol-Myers Oncology.*

276   Pazelliptine
65222-35-7

$C_{22}H_{27}N_5$
10-[[3-(Diethylamino)propyl]amino]-6-
methyl-5H-pyrido[3',4':4,5]pyrrolo-
[2,3-g]isoquinoline.
Antineoplastic agent.

277   Pegaspargase
130167-69-0   871
(Monomethoxypolyethylene glycol
succinimidyl)$_{7a}$-L-asparaginase.
Oncaspar. Antineoplastic agent. Reaction
product of asparaginase wth succinic
anhydride. Used in treatment of acute
leukemia. *Enzon, Inc.*

278   Peldesine
133432-71-0

$C_{12}H_{11}N_5O$
2-Amino-3,5-dihydro-7-(3-
pyridylmethyl)-4H-pyrrolo[3,2-d]-
pyrimidin-4-one.
BCX-34. Antineoplastic and antipsoriatic
agent. *BioCryst Pharmaceuticals, Inc.*

279   Peliomycin
1404-20-2
$C_{46}H_{76}O_{14}$
NSC-76455. Antineoplastic agent.

280   Penoctonium Bromide
17088-72-1

$C_{26}H_{50}BrNO_2$
Diethyl(2-hydroxyethyl)octyl ammonium
bromide dicyclopentylacetate.
Potential chemotherapeutic agent.

281   Pentamustine
73105-03-0

$C_8H_{16}ClN_3O_2$
1-(2-Chloroethyl)-3-neopentyl-1-
nitrosourea.
NCNU. Antineoplastic agent. *National
Foundation for Cancer Res.*

282   Pentostatin
53910-25-1   7277

$C_{11}H_{16}N_4O_4$
(R)-3-(2-Deoxy-β-D-erythro-
pentofuranosyl)-3,6,7,8-tetrahydro-
imidazo[4,5-d][1,3]diazepin-8-ol.
Co-V; Co-Vidarabine; CI-825; CL-
67310465; Covidarabine; Deaminase
inhibitor; NSC-218321; Pentostatin; PD-
ADI; Vira A deaminase inhibitor; 2'-
Dexoycoformycin; 2'-DCF; Nipent.
Antineoplastic agent. Potentiator. mp =

220-225°, 204-209.5°; λ_m = 282 nm (ε 8000 pH 7), 283 nm (ε 7970 pH 11), 283 nm (ε 7570 → 3143 over 6.5 hours pH 2); $[\alpha]_D^{25}$ = 76.4° (H_2O c = 1), $[\alpha]_D^{23}$ = 73.0° (pH 7 buffer c = 1). *Parke-Davis*.

283 Peplomycin
68247-85-8   7286

R =

$C_{61}H_{88}N_{18}O_{21}S_2$
N^1-[3-[[(S)-(α-Methylbenzyl)]amino]-propyl]bleomycinamide.
Antineoplastic agent. Bleomycin derivative with cytostatic acitvity and less pulmonary toxicity than bleomycin. *Bristol-Myers Oncology*.

284 Peplomycin Sulfate
70384-29-1   7286
$C_{61}H_{88}N_{18}O_{21}S_2 \cdot H_2SO_4$
N^1-[3-[[(S)-(α-Methylbenzyl)]amino]-propyl]bleomycinamide sulfate (1:1) (salt).
NK-631. Antineoplastic agent. Bleomycin derivative with cytostatic acitvity and less pulmonary toxicity than bleomycin. mp = 196-198°; $[\alpha]_{436}^{25}$ = -2.0° (H_2O c = 1); soluble in H_2O, MeOH, AcOH, DMSO, DMF; insoluble in less polar solvents; LD_{50} (rat sc) = 234 mg/kg, (rat ip)= 208 mg/kg, (rat iv) = 245 mg/kg, (mus sc) = 88 mg/kg, (mus ip) 85 mg/kg,. *Bristol-Myers Oncology*.

285 Perfosfamide
62435-42-1   7303

$C_7H_{15}Cl_2N_2O_4P$
($\pm$)-cis-2-[Bis(2-chloroethyl)amino]-tetrahydro-2H-1,3,2-oxazaphosphorin-4-yl hydroperoxide.
P-oxide; Pergamid; 4-HC; NSC-181815. Antineoplastic agent. mp = 107=108°; LD_{50} (rat iv) = 115 mg/kg, (rat ip) = 131 mg/kg, (mus iv) = 235 mg/kg, (mus ip) = 181 mg/kg. *Scios Nova Inc*.

286 Pipobroman
54-91-1

$C_{10}H_{16}Br_2N_2O_2$
1,4-Bis(3-bromopropionyl)-piperazine.
Amedel; N,N'-bis(3-bromopropionyl)-piperazine; Vercyte; NSC-25154; A-8103. Antineoplastic agent. *Abbott Labs*.

287 Piposulfan
2608-24-4   7635

$C_{12}H_{22}N_2O_8S_2$
1,4-Dihydracryloylpiperazine dimethanesulfonate.
A-20968; Ancyte; 1,4-Dihydracryloylpiperazine dimethane-sulfonate; NSC-47774. Antineoplastic agent. mp = 175-177°. *Abbott Labs*.

288 Pirarubicin Hydrochloride
72496-41-4   7642

$C_{32}H_{38}ClNO_{12}$
(8S,10S)-10-[[3-Amino-2,3,6-trideoxy-4-
O-(2R-tetrahydro-2H-pyran-2-yl-α-L-
lyxopyranosyl]oxy]-8-glycoloyl-7,8,9,10-
tetrahydro-6,8,11-trihydroxy-1-methoxy-
5,12-naphthacenedione.
THP-adriamycin HCl; Pirarubicin HCl;
NSC-654509. Antineoplastic agent.

289 Piritrexim
72732-56-0   7654

$C_{17}H_{19}N_5O_2$
2,4-Diamino-6-(2,5-dimethoxybenzyl)-5-
methylpyrido[2,3-d]pyrimidine.
BW-301U. Antiproliferative agent. mp =
252-254°. *Glaxo Wellcome Inc.*

290 Piritrexim Isethionate
79483-69-5   7654

$C_{17}H_{19}N_5O_2 \cdot C_2H_6O_4S$
2,4-Diamino-6-(2,5-dimethoxybenzyl)-5-
methylpyrido[2,3-d]pyrimidine mono(2-
hydroxyethanesulfonate).

BW-301U isethionate. Antiproliferative
agent. A proprietary preparation of
chlorpheniramine maleate;
antihistaminic. LD_{50} (rat orl) = 764 mg/kg;
LD_{90} (rat orl) = 1572 mg/kg. *Glaxo
Wellcome Inc.*

291 Piroxantrone
91441-23-5

$C_{21}H_{25}N_5O_4$
5-[(3-Aminopropyl)amino]-7,10-
dihydroxy-2-[2-[(2-hydroxyethyl)amino]-
ethyl]anthra[1,9-cd]pyrazol-6(2H)-one.
Antineoplastic agent. *Parke-Davis.*

292 Piroxantrone Hydrochloride
105118-12-5

$C_{21}H_{27}Cl_2N_5O_4$
5-[(3-Aminopropyl)amino]-7,10-
dihydroxy-2-[2-[(2-hydroxyethyl)amino]-
ethyl]anthra[1,9-cd]pyrazol-6(2H)-one
dihydrochloride.
CI-942. Antineoplastic agent. *Parke-
Davis.*

293 Platinol
15663-27-1   2378

$Cl_2H_6N_2Pt$
(SP-4-2)-Diamminedichloroplatinum.
cis-diamminedichloroplatinum; cis-
platinum II; cis-DDP; CACP; CPDC;
DDP; Briplatin; Cismaplat; Cisplatyl;

Citoplatino; Lederplatin; Neoplatin; Platamine; Platinex; Platiblastin; Platinol; Platinoxan; Platistin; Platosin; Rand; NSC-119875. Antineoplastic agent. mp = 270° (dec); soluble in H_2O (253 mg/100g), insoluble in organic solvents; LD_{50} (gpg ip) = 9.7 mg/kg. *Bristol-Myers Oncology.*

294   Plicamycin
18378-89-7   7696   232-455-8

$C_{22}H_{38}O_5$
[2S-[2+I,3β(1R*,3R*,4S*)]]-6-[[2,6-Dideoxy-3-O-(2,6-dideoxy-β-D-arabino-hexopyranosyl)-β-D-arabino-hexopyranosyl]oxy]-2-[(O-2,6-dideoxy-3-C-methyl-β-D-ribo-hexopyranosyl-(1→4)-O-2,6-dideoxy-α-D-lyxo-hexopyranosyl-(1→3)-2,6-dideoxy-β-D-arabino-hexopyranosyl)oxy]-3-(3,4-dihydroxy-1-methoxy-2-oxopentyl)-3,4-dihydro-8,9-dihydroxy-7-methyl-1(2H)-anthracenone.
A-2371; Antibiotic LA 7017; Aurelic acid; Aureolic acid; Mithracin; Mithramycin A; Mitramycin; PA-144; NSC-24559; plicamycin. Antineoplastic agent. mp = 180-183°; $[\alpha]_D^{20}$ = 51° (c = 0.4 EtOH); soluble in H_2O, polar organic solvents; less soluble in Et_2O, C_6H_6; LD_{50} (rat iv) = 1.74 mg/kg. *Bayer Corp., Pharmaceutical Div.*

295   Porfimer Sodium
87806-31-3   7755

Photofrin II.
CL-184116.   Antineoplastic   agent, radioprotector and radiosensitizer.

296   Porfiromycin
801-52-5   7756

$C_{16}H_{20}N_4O_5$
6-Amino-1,1a,2,8,8a,8b-hexahydro-8-(hydroxymethyl)-8a-methoxy-1,5-dimethyl-azirino[2',3':3,4]pyrrolo[1,2-a]indole-4,7-dione carbamate (ester).
Methyl mitomycin C; Methylmitomycin; N-Methylmitomycin C; Porphyromycin; NSC-56410; U-14743. Antineoplastic agent. Dec 201-202°; $[\alpha]_D^{25}$ = 275° (c = 0.1% MeOH); λ_m = 217, 360, 555 nm (ε 24600, 23000, 209 MeOH); slightly soluble in H_2O, moderately soluble in polar organic solvents; insoluble in hydrocarbon solvents. *Pharmacia & Upjohn, Inc.*

297   Prednimustine
29069-24-7   7900

$C_{35}H_{45}Cl_2NO_6$
11β,17-Dihydroxy-21-[4-[4-[bis(2-chloroethyl)amino]phenyl]-1-oxobutoxy].
Leo 1031; Sterecyt; NSC-171345; NSC-134087.   Antineoplastic   agent.
Prednisolone ester of chlorambucil. mp = 163-164°; $[\alpha]_D^{24}$ = 92.9° (CHCl$_3$ c = 1.06).
SmithKline Beecham Pharmaceuticals.

298   Procarbazine
671-16-9   7938

$C_{12}H_{19}N_3O$
N-(1-Methylethyl)-4-[(2-methyl-hydrazino)methyl]benzamide.
MIH;   Ro-4-6467;   ibenzmethyzin.
Antineoplastic agent. *Hoffmann-LaRoche Inc.*

299   Procarbazine Hydrochloride
366-70-1   7938

$C_{12}H_{20}ClN_3O$
N-(1-Methylethyl)-4-[(2-methyl-hydrazino)methyl]benzamide monohydrochloride.

NSC-77213;   Ro-4-6467/1;   ibenz-methyzin   hydrochloride;   Matulane; MBH;   MIH   hydrochloride;   PCB hydrochloride;   natulan   hydrochloride; nathulane; natulan; natulanar; IBZ; Ro-4-6467. Antineoplastic agent. mp = 223-226°; LD$_{50}$ (rat orl) = 785 mg/kg. *Hoffmann-LaRoche Inc.*

300   Proresid
1508-45-8   7703

$C_{24}H_{30}N_2O_8$
Podophyllic acid 2-ethylhydrazide.
SPI-77;   NSC-72274.   Antineoplastic agent. $[\alpha]_D$ = -154° (c = 0.5 CHCl$_3$).

301   Purinethol
50-44-2   5919   200-037-4

$C_5H_4N_4S$
1,7-Dihydro-6H-purine-6-thione.
Mercaptopurine;   Purine-6-thiol; Hypoxanthine, thio-; Ismipur; Leukeran; Leukerin;   Leupurin;   Mercaleukim; Mercaleukin; Mercapurin; Mern; Puri-Nethol; Purimethol; Purinethiol; U-4748; NSC-755; 3H-Purine-6-thiol; 6 MP; 6-Purinethiol; 6-Thioxopurine; 7-Mercapto-1,3,4,6-tetrazaindene;   6-Purinethiol hydrate;   NSC-755.   Antineoplastic, immunosuppressant. Dec 313-314°; λ_m = 230, 312 nm (ε 14000, 19600 0.1N NaOH); insoluble in H$_2$O, organic solvents; slightly soluble in EtOH; LD$_{50}$ (mus ip) = 157 mg/kg, (hamster ip) = 364 mg/kg. *Glaxo Wellcome Inc.*

302 Puromycin
53-79-2   8130

C₂₂H₂₉N₇O₅
$C_{22}H_{29}N_7O_5$
3'-(α-Amino-p-methoxyhydro-
cinnamamido)-3'-deoxy-N,N-
dimethyladenosine.
CL-16536; PDH; puromycin; X 185.
Antineoplastic, antiprotozoal
(trypanosoma) agent. mp = 175.5-177°;
$[\alpha]_D^{25}$ = -11° (EtOH); λ_m = 275 nm (ε 20300
0.13N NaOH), 267.5 nm (ε 19500 0.1N
HCl); LD$_{50}$ (mus iv) = 350 mg/kg, (mus ip)
= 525 mg/kg; (mus orl) = 675 mg/kg. *ICN
Pharmaceuticals, Inc.*

303 Puromycin Hydrochloride
58-58-2   8130

$C_{22}H_{31}Cl_2N_7O_5$
3'-(α-Amino-p-methoxyhydro-
cinnamamido)-3'-deoxy-N,N-
dimethyladenosine dihydrochloride.
CL-13900 dihydrochloride; P-638
dihydrochloride; Stylomycin dihydrochloride; 3123L, dihydrochloride; NSC-
3055. Antineoplastic, antiprotozoal
(trypanosoma) agent. *ICN
Pharmaceuticals, Inc.*

304 Pyrazofurin
30868-30-5

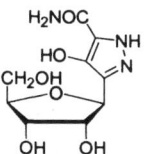

$C_9H_{13}N_3O_6$
4-Hydroxy-3-β-D-ribofuranosylpyrazole-
5-carboxamide.
4-hydroxy-3-β-D-ribofuranosyl-1H-
pyrazole-5-carboxamide; NSC-143095;
Pirazofurin; β-Pyrazomycin;
Pyrazomycin; Pyrozofurin; Przf;
Pyrazofurin; Pyrazomycin; 47599.
Antineoplastic agent. *Eli Lilly & Co.*

305 Raltitrexed
112887-68-0   9684

$C_{21}H_{22}N_4O_6S$
N-[5-[[3,4-Dihydro-2-methyl-4-oxo-6-
quinazolinyl)methyl]methylamino]-2-
thenoyl]-L-glutamic acid.
Tomudex; ZD-1694. Antineoplastic
agent. Thymidylate synthase inhibitor,
used in treatment of advanced colorectal
cancer. Monohydrate is soluble in H$_2$O,
mp = 180-184°. *Zeneca Pharmaceuticals.*

306 (±)-Razoxane
21416-87-5   8295

$C_{11}H_{16}N_4O_4$
4,4'-(1-Methyl-1,2-ethanediyl)bis-2,6-
piperazinedione.
Razoxin; (±)-4,4'-propylenedi-2,6-pipera-

zinedione; (±)-(3,5,3',5'-tetraoxo)-1,2-dipiperazinopropane; ICI-59118; ICRF-159; NSC-129943. Razoxin is an anticancer preparation containing razoxane. mp = 237-239°. *ICI Chemicals and Polymers Ltd.*

307   Regamycin
801-52-5   7756

$C_{16}H_{20}N_4O_5$
6-Amino-1,1a,2,8,8a,8b-hexahydro-8-(hydroxymethyl)-8a-methoxy-1,5-dimethyl-azirino[2',3':3,4]pyrrolo[1,2-a]-indole-4,7-dione carbamate (ester).
Methyl mitomycin C; Methylmitomycin; N-Methylmitomycin C; Porphyromycin; NSC-56410; U-14743. Antineoplastic agent. Dec 201-202°; $[\alpha]_D^{25}$ = 275° (c = 0.1% MeOH); λ_m = 217, 360, 555 nm (ε 24600, 23000, 209 MeOH); slightly soluble in H_2O, moderately soluble in polar organic solvents, insoluble in hydrocarbon solvents. *Pharmacia & Upjohn, Inc.*

308   Retelliptine
72238-02-9

$C_{25}H_{42}N_4O$
1-[[3-(Diethylamino)propyl]amino]-9-methoxy-5,11-dimethyl-6H-pyrido-[4,3-b]carbazole.
Antineoplastic agent.

309   Retin-A
302-79-4   8333   206-129-0

$C_{20}H_{28}O_2$
all-trans-Retinoic acid.
Tretinoin 25WM; Vesanoid; NSC-122758. Keratolytic. Has antineoplastic activity. mp = 180-181°; λ_m = 351 nm (ε 45000 MeOH); LD_{50} (rat orl 10 day) = 2000 mg/kg. *BASF Corp; Hoffmann-LaRoche Inc.; Ortho Pharmaceutical Corp.*

310   Riboprine
7724-76-7

$C_{15}H_{21}N_5O_4$
N-(3-Methyl-2-butenyl)adenosine.
IPA; NSC-105546. Antineoplastic agent. *Roswell Park Memorial Inst.*

311   Rituximab
174722-31-7
Immunoglobulin G1 disulfide with human-mouse monoclonal IDEC-C2B8 kappa-chain, dimer.
IDEC-C2B8; IDEC-102. Antineoplastic agent. Microtubule inhibitor. *IDEC Pharmaceuticals Corp.*

312   Rodorubicin
96497-67-5

$C_{48}H_{64}N_2O_{17}$
(1S,3R,4R)-3-Ethyl-1,2,3,4,6,11-
hexahydro-3,5,10,12-tetrahydroxy-6,11-
dioxo-4-[[2,3,6-trideoxy-3-(dimethylamino)-α-L-lyxohexo-pyranosyl]oxy]-1-
naphthacenyl   O-3,6-dideoxy-α-L-eryth-
rohexopyranos-4-ulosyl(1→4)-O-2,6-
dideoxy-α-L-lyxohexopyranosyl(1→4)-
2,3,6-trideoxy-3-(dimethylamino)-α-L-
lyxohexo-pyranoside 2,3'-anhydride.
Antineoplastic agent.

313   Rogletimide
121840-95-7

$C_{12}H_{14}N_2O_2$
(±)-2-Ethyl-2-(4-pyridyl)glutarimide.
Antineoplastic agent. U.S. Bioscience.

314   Safingol
15639-50-6

$C_{18}H_{39}NO_2$
(2S,3S)-2-Amino-1,3-octadecanediol.
Antineoplastic, antipsoriatic agent.
Sphinx Pharmaceutical Corp.

315   Safingol Hydrochloride
139755-79-6

$C_{18}H_{40}ClNO_2$
(2S,3S)-2-Amino-1,3-octadecanediol
hydrochloride.
Antineoplastic, antipsoriatic agent.
Sphinx Pharmaceutical Corp.

316   Samarium Sm-153 Lexidronam Pentasodium
154427-83-5

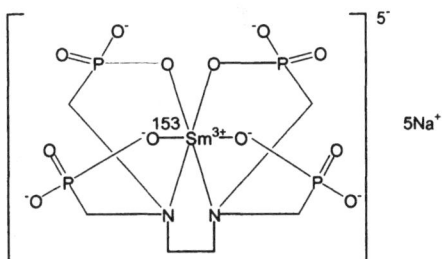

$C_6H_{17}N_2O_{12}P_4^{153}Sm$
[N,N'O^P,OP;ks',O^{P_I},o$^{P_{III}}$]-[[[1,2-ethane-
diylbis[nitrilobis(methylene)]]tetrakis-
[phosphonato]](8-)-Samarate-(5-)-^{153}Sm.
Antineoplastic agent. Cytogen Corp.

317   Sedoxantrone Trihydrochloride
119221-49-7

$C_{21}H_{30}Cl_3N_5OS$
5-[(2-Aminoethyl)amino]-2-[2-
(diethylamino)ethyl]-2H-[1]-
benzothiopyrano[4,3,2-cd]indazol-8-ol
trihydrochloride.
CI-958. Antineoplastic agent. DNA
topoisomerase II inhibitor. Parke-Davis.

318   Semustine
13909-09-6

C_{10}H_{18}ClN_{3}O_{2}
1-(2-Chloroethyl)-3-(4-methyl-cyclohexyl)-1-nitrosourea.
methyl CCNU; trans-Methyl-CCNU; Lomustine, methyl; MeCCNU; NSC-95441. Antineoplastic agent.

319   Sendoxan
6055-19-2   2816

C_{7}H_{15}Cl_{2}N_{2}O_{2}P.H_{2}O
N,N-Bis(2-Chloroethyl)tetrahydro-2H-1,3,2-oxazaphosphorin-2-amine 2-oxide.
2-[bis(2-chloroethyl)amino]tetrahydro-2H-1,3,2-oxazophosphorine 2-oxide; 1-bis-(2-chloroethyl)amino-1-oxa-2-aza-5-oxaphosphoridin; B 518; Cycloblastin; Cyclostin; Endoxan; Procytox; Sendoxan; Cytoxan; NSC-26271. Antineoplastic agent. mp = 41°; soluble in H_{2}O (10-50 mg/ml), poorly soluble in organic solvents; LD_{50} (rat orl) = 94 mg/kg. *Degussa AG.*

320   Simtrazene
5579-27-1

C_{14}H_{16}N_{4}
1,4-Dimethyl-1,4-diphenyl-2-tetrazene.
CL-26193; NSC-83799. Antineoplastic agent.

321   Sobuzoxane
98631-95-9   8708

C_{22}H_{34}N_{4}O_{10}
4,4'-Ethylenebis[1-(hydroxymethyl)-2,6-piperazinedione] bis(isobutyl carbonate).
Antineoplastic agent. mp = 128-130°, 132-133°; insoluble in H_{2}O; LD_{50} (mmus ip) = 807 mg/kg, (mmus sc) = 400 mg/kg, (fmus ip) = 960 mg/kg, (fmus sc) = 673 mg/kg, (mrat ip)= 877 mg/kg, (mrat sc) = 3025 mg/kg, (frat ip) = 567 mg/kg, (frat sc) = 2821 mg/kg; reported as >5000 mg/kg orl in all species.

322   Sodium Phenylbutyrate
1716-12-7

C_{10}H_{11}NaO_{2}
Sodium 4-phenylbutyrate.
PBA; Buphenyl; TriButyrate. A short-chain aromatic fatty acid that inhibits cell proliferation and induces apoptosis. Also used in treatment of ornithine transcarbamylase deficiency as a vehicle for waste nitrogen excretion in patients with inborn errors of urea synthesis. Antineoplastic, hematopoietic and antihyperammonemic. Used to reduce levels of ammonia in the blood.

323 Sparfosate Sodium
66569-27-5

$$HOOC-\overset{H}{\underset{NHCOCH_2PO(ONa)_2}{|}}-CH_2COOH$$

$C_6H_8NNa_2O_8P$
N-(Phosphonoacetyl)-L-aspartic acid
disodium salt.
CI-882. Antineoplastic agent. *Parke-Davis*.

324 Sparfosic Acid
51321-79-0

$$HOOC-\overset{H}{\underset{NHCOCH_2PO(OH)_2}{|}}-CH_2COOH$$

$C_6H_{10}NO_8P$
N-(Phosphonoacetyl)-L-aspartic acid.
Antineoplastic agent. *Parke-Davis*.

325 Spirogermanium
41992-23-8   8916

$C_{17}H_{38}Cl_2GeN_2$
2-[3-(Dimethylamino)propyl]-8,8-diethyl-
2-aza-8-germaspiro[4.5]decane
dihydrochloride.
Spirogermanium 32. Antineoplastic
agent. Cytostatic germanium derivative.
mp = 287-288°; LD_{50} (mus orl) = 324
mg/kg. *Unimed, Inc.*

326 Spirogermanium Dihydrochloride
41992-22-7   8916

$C_{17}H_{36}GeN_2$
2-[3-(Dimethylamino)propyl]-8,8-diethyl-
2-aza-8-germaspiro[4.5]decane.
spirogermanium; Spiro-32; NSC-192965.

Antineoplastic agent. mp = 287-288°;
LD_{50} (mus orl) = 324 mg/kg. *Unimed, Inc.*

327 Spiromustine
56605-16-4

$C_{14}H_{23}Cl_2N_3O_2$
3-[2-[Bis(2-chloroethyl)amino]ethyl]-1,3-
diazaspiro[4.5]decane-2,4-dione.
Spirohydantoin mustard; SHM; NSC-
172112. Antineoplastic agent.

328 Spiroplatin
74790-08-2

$C_8H_{18}N_2O_4PtS$
cis[1,1-Cyclohexanebis(methylamine)]-
(sulfato)platinum.
NSC-311056. Antineoplastic agent.
Bristol-Myers Oncology.

329 ST 52
522-40-7   4279   208-328-8

$C_{18}H_{22}O_8P_2$
Diethylstilbestrol bisphosphate.
DESDP; α,α'-diethyl-(E)-4,4'-stilbenediol
bis(dihydrogen phosphate); NSC-10481;
diethylstilbestryl bisphosphate; fosfestrol;
honvan; phosphestrol; ST52-Asta;
stilbestrol bisphosphate; stilphostrol;
fosfesterol. Antineoplastic (hormonal);
estrogen. mp = 204-206° (dec); poorly
soluble in H_2O.

330 Streptonigrin
3930-19-6 8986 223-501-8

$C_{25}H_{22}N_4O_8$
5-Amino-6-(7-amino-5,8-dihydro-6-methoxy-5,8-dioxo-2-quinolyl)-4-(2-hydroxy-3,4-dimethoxyphenyl)-3-methyl-2-pyridinecarboxylic acid.
streptoniazide; Strazide; Streptohydrazid; Nigrin; NSC-45383; A 050165L302; Abbott Crystalline antibiotic; Bruneomycin; Nigrin; Rufochromomycin; Rufocromomycin; Streptonigran; STP; 5278 R. P. Antineoplastic agent. Antitumor antibiotic from *Streptomyces flocculus*. mp = 262-263°; dec 275°; λ_m = 248, 375-380 nm (ε 38400, 17400 MeOH); slightly soluble in H_2O, more soluble in polar organic solvents. *Pfizer Inc.*

331 Streptozocin
18883-66-4 8991

$C_8H_{15}N_3O_7$
2-Deoxy-2-[[(methylnitrosoamino)-carbonyl]amino]-D-glucose.
NSC-85998; Streptozoticin; Streptozotocin, Pure; STZ; U-9889; Zanosar. Antineoplastic agent. mp= 115° (dec); soluble in H_2O, lower alcohols, ketones; λ_m = 228 nm (ε 6360); LD_{50} (mus ip) = 360 mg/kg. *Pharmacia & Upjohn, Inc.*

332 Sufosfamide
37753-10-9

$C_8H_{18}ClN_2O_5PS$
2-[[3-(2-Chloroethyl)tetrahydro-2H-1,3,2-oxazaphosphorin-2-yl]amino]-ethanol methanesulfonate (ester).
An oxazaphosphorine derivative. Antineoplastic; immunosuppressant.

333 Sulofenur
110311-27-8

$C_{16}H_{15}ClN_2O_3S$
1-(p-Chlorophenyl)-3-(5-indanylsulfonyl)-urea.
LY-186641. Antineoplastic agent. *Eli Lilly & Co.*

334 Sunfural®
17902-23-7 9267

$C_8H_9FN_2O_3$
5-Fluoro-1-(tetrahydro-2-furanyl)-2,4(1H,3H)-pyrimidinedione.
Tegafur; FT-207; MJF-12264; Citofur; Coparogin; Exonal; Fental; NSC-148958; Franrose; Ftorafur; Fulaid; Fulfeel; Furafluor; Furofutran; Futraful; Lamar; Lifril; Neberk; Nitobanil; Riol; Sinoflurol; Tefsiel C. Antineoplastic agent. mp = 164-165°; λ_m = 270 nm (ε 8460 pH 2, 8050 pH 7, 6700 pH 12); soluble in H_2O, EtOH, DMF, insoluble in Et_2O; LD_{50} (mus orl 3 day) = 900 mg/kg, (mus orl) = 750 mg/kg, (mus ip) = 1150 mg/kg. *Asahi Chem. Industry.*

335 Sunrabin®
55726-47-1 3624

$C_{31}H_{55}N_3O_6$
N-(1-β-D-Arabinofuranosyl-1,2-dihydro-2-oxo-4-pyrimidinyl)docosanamide.
enocitabine; NSC-239336. Antineoplastic agent. mp = 141-142°; $[\alpha]_D$ = 70° (THF, c = 1.0, 22°); λ_m = 216, 248, 303 nm (ε 16400, 15200, 8200).

336 Tabloid
154-42-7 9473 205-827-2

$C_5H_5N_5S.xH_2O$
2-Aminopurine-6(1H)-thione.
thioguanine; tioguanine; NSC-752. Antineoplastic agent. mp > 360°. *Glaxo Wellcome Inc.*

337 Tallimustine
115308-98-0
$C_{32}H_{38}Cl_2N_{10}O_4$
N-(2-Amidinoethyl)-4-[p-[bis(2-chloroethyl)amino]benzamido]-1,1',1-trimethyl-N,4':N',4-ter[pyrrole-2-carboxamide.
PNU-152241; FCE-24517. Distamycin-A derivative. Antineoplastic; antitumor.

338 Tamoxifen
10540-29-1 9216

$C_{26}H_{29}NO$
(Z)-2-[p-(1,2-Diphenyl-1-butenyl)-phenoxy]-N,N-dimethylamine.
Antineoplastic agent; antiestrogen. Nonsteroidal estrogen antagonist. mp = 96-98°. *ICI.*

339 Tamoxifen Citrate
54965-24-1 9216

$C_{26}H_{29}NO.C_6H_8O_7$
(Z)-2-[p-(1,2-Diphenyl-1-butenyl)-phenoxy]-N,N-dimethylamine citrate.
ICI-46474; Nolvadex; Tamoxifen; Tamoxifen citrate; TMX; NSC-180973. Antineoplastic agent; antiestrogen. mp = 140-142°; slightly soluble in H_2O; more soluble in EtOH, MeOH, Me_2CO; LD_{50} (mus ip) = 200 mg/kg, (mus iv) = 62.5 mg/kg, (mus orl) = 3000-6000 mg/kg, (rat ip) = 600 mg/kg), (rat iv) = 62.5 mg/kg, (rat orl) = 1200-2500 mg/kg. *ICI.*

340 Tauromustine
85977-49-7

$C_7H_{15}ClN_4O_4S$
1-(2-Chloroethyl)-3-[2-(dimethyl-sulfamoyl)ethyl]-1-nitrosourea.
TCNU. Chemotherapeutic; antitumor.

341 Tecogalan Sodium
134633-29-7
DS-4152. Antineoplastic agent (adjunct).
Fermentation product of *Arthrobacter* sp.
AT-25. *Daiichi Pharmaceutical Corp.*

342 Tegafur
17902-23-7   9267

$C_8H_9FN_2O_3$
5-Fluoro-1-(tetrahydro-2-furanyl)-
2,4(1H,3H)-pyrimidinedione.
Sunfural; FT-207; MJF-12264; Citofur;
Coparogin; Exonal; Fental; NSC-148958;
Franrose; Ftorafur; Fulaid; Fulfeel;
Furafluor; Furofutran; Futraful; Lamar;
Lifril; Neberk; Nitobanil; Riol; Sinoflurol;
Tefsiel C. Antineoplastic agent. mp =
164-165°; λ_m = 270 nm (ε 8460 pH 2,
8050 pH 7, 6700 pH 12); soluble in
H_2O, EtOH, DMF; insoluble in Et_2O; LD_{50}
(mus orl 3 day) = 900 mg/kg, (mus orl) =
750 mg/kg, (mus ip) = 1150 mg/kg. *Asahi
Chem. Industry.*

343 Teloxantrone
91441-48-4

$C_{23}H_{29}N_5O_6$
7,10-Dihydroxy-2-[2-[(2-hydroxyethyl)-

amino]ethyl]-5-[[2-(methylamino)ethyl]-
amino]-anthra[1,9-cd]pyrazol-6(2H)-one
acetate (salt) hydrobromide (10:5:21).
Moxantrazole; DUP-937; NSC-355644.
Antineoplastic agent. *DuPont Merck
Pharmaceutical Co.*

344 Teloxantrone Hydrochloride
132937-88-3

$C_{23}H_{30}ClN_5O_6$
7,10-Dihydroxy-2-[2-[(2-hydroxyethyl)-
amino]ethyl]-5-[[2-(methylamino)ethyl]-
amino]anthra[1,9-cd]pyrazol-6(2H)-one
acetate (salt) hydrobromide (10:5:21)
hydroxide.
NSC-355644. Antineoplastic agent.
DuPont Merck Pharmaceutical Co.

345 Temoporfin
122341-38-2

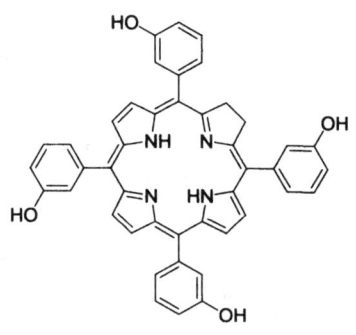

$C_{44}H_{32}N_4O_4$
3,3',3,3''''-(7,8-Dihydroporphyrin-
5,10,15,20-tetrayl)tetraphenol.
EF9. Antineoplastic agent. *Scotia
Pharmaceuticals, Ltd.*

346 Temozolomide
85622-93-1   9289

$C_6H_6N_6O_2$
3,4-Dihydro-3-methyl-4-oxoimidazo-[5,1-d]-as-tetrazine-8-carboxamide.
M&B-39831; Methazolastone; NSC-362856. Antineoplastic agent. mp = 212° (dec); λ_m = 327 nm (EtOH). *May & Baker Ltd.*

347 Teniposide
29767-20-2   9291

$C_{32}H_{32}O_{13}S$
[5R-[5α,5aβ,8aα,9β(R*)]]-5,8,8a,9-Tetrahydro-5-(4-hydroxy-3,5-dimethoxyphenyl)-9-[[4,6-O-(2-thienylmethylene)-β-D-glucopyranosyl]oxy]furo[3',4':6,7]-naphtho[2,3-d]-1,3-dioxol-6(5aH)-one.
ETP; VM-26; Vehem-Sandoz; Vumon; NSC-362856; 4'-demethylepipodo-phyllotoxin-β-D-thenylidine glucoside; 4'-demethylepipodo-phyllotoxin 9-(4,6-O-2-thenylidene-β-D-glucopyranoside).
Antineoplastic agent. Semi-synthetic derivative of podophyllotoxin. mp = 242-246°; $[\alpha]_D^{20}$ = -107° (CHCl$_3$/MeOH, 9:1); λ_m = 283 nm (E$_{1cm}^{1\%}$ 64.1, MeOH); pKa = 10.3. *Sandoz Pharmaceuticals Corp.*

348 Teroxirone
59653-73-5

$C_{12}H_{15}N_3O_6$
(RS,RS,SR)-1,3,5-Tris(2,3-epoxypropyl)-s-triazine-2,4,6(1H,3H,5H)-trione.
α-triglycidyl isocyanurate; αTGI; NSC-296934. Antineoplastic agent.

349 Teslac
968-93-4   9321   213-534-6

$C_{19}H_{24}O_3$
13-Hydroxy-3-oxo-13,17-secoandrosta-1,4-dien-17-oic acid δ-lactone.
testolactone; SQ-9538; Fludestrin; NSC-12173; NSC-23759. Antineoplastic agent. mp = 218-219°; $[\alpha]_D^{23}$ = -46° (c = 1.24 CHCl$_3$); λ_m = 242 nm (ε 15800, EtOH). *Bristol-Myers Oncology.*

350 Theriodide I-131
7790-26-3   8778

$$Na^{+\ 131}I^-$$

^{131}INa
Sodium iodide-^{131}I.
Antineoplastic, radioactive agent. Radioactive iodine (^{131}I) is a β- and σ-emitter with a halflife of 8 days. *Abbott Labs.*

351   Thiamiprine
5581-52-2   9434

$C_9H_8N_8O_2S$
2-Amino-6-[(1-methyl-4-nitro-1H-imidazol-5-yl)thio]purine.
BW-57-323; Guaneran; NSC-38887. Antineoplastic agent. mp > 200° (dec); λ_m = 320 nm (pH 1), 315 nm (pH 11). *Glaxo Wellcome Inc.*

352   Thioguanine Hemihydrate
5580-03-0

$C_5H_5N_5S.xH_2O$
2-Amino-1,7-dihydro-6H-purine-6-thione.
Lanvis; BW-5071; Tabloid; Thioguanine; Tioguanin; Tioguanine; TG; Wellcome U3B; X 27; NSC-752. mp > 360°.

353   Thiotepa
52-24-4   9805   200-135-7

$C_6H_{12}N_3PS$
1,1',1''-Phosphinothioylidynetris-aziridine.
CBC-806495; Girostan; NCI-C01649; Oncotepa; Oncothio-tepa; SK-6882; STEPA; Tespa; NSC-6396; Tespamin; Tespamine; Thio-tepa; Thio-tepa S; Thio-Tep; Thio-Tepa; Thiofozil; Thiotef; Thiotepa; Thioplex; Tifosyl; Tio-tef; Tiofosfamid; Tiofosyl; Tiofozil; TESPA; TIO TEF; TSPA. Antineoplastic agent. mp = 51°; soluble in H_2O (190 g/l), organic

solvents; LD_{50} (rat iv) = 15 mg/kg. *Immunex Corp.*

354   Thymalfasin
62304-98-7
$C_{129}H_{215}N_{33}O_{55}$
N-Acetyl-L-seryl-L-α-aspartyl-L-alanyl-L-alanyl-L-valyl-L-α-aspartyl-L-threonyl-L-seryl-L-seryl-L-α-glutamyl-L-isoleucyl-L-threonyl-L-threonyl-L-lysyl-L-α-aspartyl-L-leucyl-L-lysyl-L-α-glutamyl-L-lysyl-L-lysyl-L-α-glutamyl-L-valyl-L-valyl-L-α-glutamyl-L-α-glutamyl-L-alanyl-L-α-glutamyl-L-asparagine.
thymosin-α1; Zadaxin. Antineoplastic. Also used in hepatitis treatment, vaccine enhancement, treatment of infec-tious diseases. *SciClone Pharmaceuticals, Inc.*

355   Tiazofurin
60084-10-8

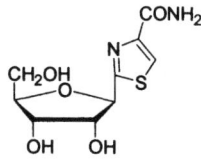

$C_9H_{12}N_2O_5S$
2-β-D-Ribofuranosyl-4-thiazolecarboxamide.
CI-909; NSC-286193. Antineoplastic agent. *Parke-Davis.*

356   Tirapazamine
27314-97-2

$C_7H_6N_4O_2$
3-Amino-1,2,4-benzotriazine 1,4-dioxide.
WIN-59075; SR-4233; Triazone; SR-259075. Antineoplastic agent. A hypoxic cytotoxin, used in combination with cisplatin.

357 Topotecan
123948-87-8   9687

C$_{23}$H$_{23}$N$_3$O$_5$
(S)-10-[(Dimethylamino)methyl]-4-ethyl-4,9-dihydroxy-1H-pyrano[3',4':6,7]-indolizino[1,2-b]quinoline-3,14(4H,12H)-dione.
Antineoplastic agent. DNA topoisomerase I inhibitor. soluble in H$_2$O (< 1 mg/ml). *SmithKline Beecham Pharmaceuticals.*

358 Topotecan Hydrochloride
119413-54-6   9687

C$_{23}$H$_{24}$ClN$_3$O$_5$
(S)-10-[(Dimethylamino)methyl]-4-ethyl-4,9-dihydroxy-1H-pyrano[3',4':6,7]-indolizino[1,2-b]quinoline-3,14(4H,12H)-dione monohydrochloride.
SK&FS-104864-A. Antineoplastic agent. DNA topoisomerase I inhibitor. *SmithKline Beecham Pharmaceuticals.*

359 Tracervial-131
7790-26-3   8778
^{131}INa
Sodium iodide-^{131}I.

Antineoplastic, radioactive agent. Radioactive iodine (^{131}I) is a β- and σ-emitter with a half-life of 8 days. *Abbott Labs.*

360 Trenimon
68-76-8   9733   200-692-6

C$_{12}$H$_{13}$N$_3$O$_2$
2,3,5-Tris(1-aziridinyl)-2,5-cyclohexadiene-1,4-dione.
A 163; Bayer 3231; Oncoredox; Oncovedex; Prenimon; Riker 601; Treninon; NSC-29215; Triaziquinone; Triaziquon; Triaziquone; triethylen-iminobenzoquinone; tris(aziridinyl)-p-benzoquinone; TEIB; 10257 R.P. Antineoplastic agent. mp = 162-163°; poorly soluble in H$_2$O, soluble in oganic solvents. *Bayer Corp., Pharmaceutical Div.*

361 Triaziquone
68-76-8   9733   200-692-6

C$_{12}$H$_{13}$N$_3$O$_2$
2,3,5-Tris(1-aziridinyl)-2,5-cyclohexadiene-1,4-dione.
A 163; Bayer 3231; Oncoredox; Oncovedex; Prenimon; Riker 601; Trenimon; Treninon; NSC-29215; Triaziquinone; Triaziquon; triethylen-iminobenzoquinone; tris(aziridinyl)-p-benzoquinone; TEIB; 10257 R.P. Antineoplastic agent. mp = 162-163°; poorly soluble in H$_2$O, soluble in oganic solvents. *Bayer Corp., Pharmaceutical Div.*

362 Trichlormethine
555-77-1 9777

$C_6H_{12}Cl_3N$
2,2',2-Trichlorotriethylamine.
trimustine; Hn3; Lekamin; R 47; Sinalost; SK-100; Trichlormethine; Trillekamin; Trimitan; Trimustine; NSC-260424; Tris-N-lost; TS-160; tris(β-chloroethyl)amine. Antineoplastic agent [as hydrochloride]. CAUTION: vesicant and necrotizing irritant. Liquid; mp= -4°; bp_{15} = 144°; d_4^{25}= 1.2347; slightly soluble in H_2O, soluble in organic solvents; miscible with many organic solvents and oils.

363 Triciribine Phosphate
61966-08-3

$C_3H_4Cl_3NO_2$
2,2,2-Trichloroethanol carbamate.
Compralgyl; trichloroethyl urethan; 2,2,2-trichloroethyl carbamate; carbamic acid trichloroethyl ester; Voluntal. Antineoplastic agent. *Bayer Corp., Pharmaceutical Div.*

364 Triethylenemelamine
51-18-3 9803

$C_9H_{12}N_6$
2,4,6-Tris(1-aziridinyl)-1,3,5-triazine.
DRP-859025; ENT-25296; M-9500; Persistol; Persistol HOE-1/193; R-246; SK-1133; NSC-9706; Tem-Simes; Tretamin; Tretamine; Triamelin; Triaziridinyl triazine; Triethano-melamine; Triethylenemelamine; Tris(ethyleneimino)triazine; Trisaziri-dinyltriazine; TAT; TEM; TET. Antineoplastic agent. mp = 39° (dec); soluble in H_2O (40%), less soluble in organic solvents; LD_{50} (mus ip) = 2.8 mg/kg, (mus orl) = 15 mg/kg, (rat ip) = 1.0 mg/kg, (rat orl) = 13 mg/kg.

365 Trimetrexate
52128-35-5 9851

$C_{19}H_{23}N_5O_3$
5-Methyl-6-[[(3,4,5-trimethoxyphenyl)-amino]methyl]-2,4-quinazolinediamine.
TMQ; CI-898; NSC-249008. Antineoplastic agent. *Parke-Davis.*

366 Trimetrexate Glucuronate
82952-64-5   9851

$C_{25}H_{33}N_5O_{10}$
5-Methyl-6-[[(3,4,5-trimethoxyphenyl)-amino]methyl]-2,4-quinazolinediamine mono-D-glucuronate.
NSC-249008. Antineoplastic agent. Soluble in H_2O (> 50 mg/ml). Parke-Davis.

367 Trofosfamide
22089-22-1   9897

$C_9H_{18}Cl_3N_2O_2P$
N,N,3-Tris(2-chloroethyl)tetrahydro-2H-1,3,2-oxazaphosphorin-2-amine 2-oxide. Z-4828; Ixoten; trilophosphamide; NSC-109723. Antineoplastic agent. mp = 50-51°; $[\alpha]_D^{25}$ = -28.6° (MeOH, c = 2.0); LD_{50} (mus ip) = 212 mg/kg. Asta-Werke AG.

368 Tubulozole
84697-22-3

$C_{23}H_{23}Cl_2N_3O_4S$
Ethyl (±)-cis-p-[[[2-(2,4-dichlorophenyl)-2-(imidazol-1-ylmethyl)-1,3-dioxolan-4-yl]methyl]thio]carbanilate.

R-46846; NSC-376450. Antineoplastic agent. Microtubule inhibitor. Janssen Pharmaceutical, Belgium.

369 Tubulozole Hydrochloride
83529-08-2

$C_{23}H_{24}Cl_3N_3O_4S$
Ethyl (±)-cis-p-[[[2-(2,4-dichlorophenyl)-2-(imidazol-1-ylmethyl)-1,3-dioxolan-4-yl]methyl]thio]carbanilate monohydrochloride.
NSC-376450; R-46846. Antineoplastic agent. microtubule inhibitor. Janssen Pharmaceutica, Belgium.

370 Turosteride
137099-09-3

$C_{27}H_{45}N_3O_3$
1-(4-Methyl-3-oxo-4-aza-5 alpha-androstane-17 beta-carbonyl)-1,3-diisopropylurea.
FCE-26073. A potent and selective inhibitor of 5 alpha-reductase, the enzyme responsible for the conversion of testosterone to 5 alpha-dihydrotestosterone. Antineoplastic; antitumor agent.

371   Ubenimex
58970-76-6   9973

$C_{16}H_{24}N_2O_4$
(-)-N-[(2S,3R)-3-Amino-2-hydroxy-4-phenylbutyryl]-L-leucine.
Bestatin;   NK-421;   NSC-265489.
Antineoplastic agent; immunomodulator.
Dipeptide antitumor antibiotic produced by   *Streptomyces   olivoreticuli.*
Competitive inhibitor of aminopepptidast B and leucine aminopeptidease. mp = 233-236°; $[\alpha]_D^{w20}$ = -15.5° (1N HCl c = 1.0); λ_m =241.5, 248, 253, 258. 264.5, 268 nm ($E_{1\ cm}^{1\%}$ 3.8, 4.0, 5.0, 6.0, 4.6, 2.7); soluble in polar organic solvents; insoluble in hexane, ethyl acetate, $CHCl_3$, C_6H_6; LD_{50} (14 day) (mus sc) = 1.3-1.9 g/kg, (mus ip) = 0.19 g/kg, (mus orl) > 4.0 g/kg, (rat ip) = 1.9-2.1 g/kg, (rat sc) = 0.78-0.90 g/kg, (rat orl) > 2.0 g/kg.

372   Uracil Mustard
66-75-1   9986   200-631-3

$C_8H_{11}Cl_2N_3O_2$
5-[Bis(2-chloroethyl)amino]uracil.
U-8344;   Aminouracil   mustard; Chlorethaminacil;   CB-4835; Demethyldopan; Desmethyldopan; NSC-34462; ENT 50439; Nordopan; NCI-C04820; NSC-34462; SK-19849; U 8344; U-8344; Uracil nitrogen mustard; Uracillost; Uracilmostaza; Uramustin; Uramustine. Antineoplastic agent. mp = 206° (dec); slightly soluble in H_2O; λ_m = 257 nm (ε 5675, 0.01N H_2SO_4 in 95% EtOH); LD_{50} (rat ip)= 1.25-2.5 mg/kg.

373   Uredepa
302-49-8   10011

$C_7H_{14}N_3O_3P$
Ethyl [bis(1-aziridinyl)phosphinyl]-carbamate.
Avinar; AB 100; AB-100; bis(ethylen-imido)phosphorylurethan; NSC-37095. Antineoplastic agent. mp = 88-90°; soluble in H_2O. *Armour Pharmaceuticals.*

374   Urethane
51-79-6   10013

$C_3H_7NO_2$
Ethyl carbamate.
ethyl urethan; NSC-746. Antineoplastic agent. mp = 48-50°; bp = 182-184°; soluble in H_2O (2 g/ml), soluble in organic solvents; MLD (mus ip) = 2.1-2.2 g/kg.

375   Valspodar
121584-18-7

Ala-D-Ala-MeLeu-MeLeu-MeVal-N──────Val-MeGly-MeLeu-Val-MeLeu

$C_{63}H_{111}N_{11}O_{12}$
Cyclo[[(2S,4R,6E)-4-methyl-2-(methylamino)-3-oxo-6-octenoyl]-L-valyl-N-methylglycyl-N-methyl-L-leucyl-L-valyl-N-methyl-L-leucyl-L-alanyl-D-alanyl-N-methyl-L-leucyl-N-methyl-L-valyl].
PSC-833;   Amdray.   Third-generation cyclosporine analog, an inhibitor of P-glycoprotein, the drug efflux pump.

Multidrug resistance modulator coadministered with chemotherapeutic drugs in cancer treatment. Chemosensitizer. *Sandoz Pharmaceuticals Corp.*

376   Vapreotide
103222-11-3

$C_{57}H_{70}N_{12}O_9S_2$
D-Phenylalanyl-L-cysteinyl-L-tyrosyl-D-tryptophyl-L-lysyl-L-valyl-L-cysteinyl-L-tryptophanamide cyclic (2-7) disulfide. RC-160; BMY-41606. Antineoplastic agent. *Bristol-Myers Squibb Pharmaceutical Res. and Dev.*

377   Velban
143-67-9   10119 205-606-0

$C_{46}H_{60}N_4O_{13}S$
Vincaleukoblastine sulfate.
vinblastine sulfate; 29060-LE; Velsar; Belvan, VLB; Exal; Vincaleukoblastine sulfate (1:1) (salt); VLB monosulfate; Velbe; NSC-49842. Antineoplastic agent. mp = 284-285°; $[\alpha]_D^{26}$ = -28° (c = 1.01 in MeOH). *Eli Lilly & Co.*

378   Velbe
143-67-9   10119
$C_{46}H_{60}N_4O_{13}S$
Vincaleukoblastine sulfate.
vinblastine sulfate; 29060-LE; Velsar;

Belvan, VLB; Exal; Vincaleukoblastine sulfate (1:1) (salt); VLB monosulfate; Velban; NSC-49842. Antineoplastic agent. mp = 284-285°; $[\alpha]_D^{26}$ = -28° (c = 1.01 in MeOH). *Eli Lilly & Co.*

379   Vepesid
33419-42-0   3931

$C_{29}H_{32}O_{13}$
[5R-[5α,5aβ,8aα,9β(R*)]]-9-[(4,6-O-Ethylidene-β-D-glucopyranosyl)oxy]-5,8,8a,9-tetrahydro-5-(4-hydroxy-3,5-dimethoxyphenyl)-furo[3',4':6,7]-naphtho[2,3-d]-1,3-dioxol-6(5aH)-one. Toposar; VP-16-213; NSC-141540; Demethy-epipodophyllotoxin,ethylidene glucoside; Epipodophyllotoxin VP-16213; Etoposide; EPE; etoposide; Vepesid; Vepesid J; VP 16-213; VP-16. mp = 236-251°; $[\alpha]_D^{20}$ = -110.5° (c = 0.6 in CHCl$_3$). *Bristol-Myers Oncology.*

380   Vercyte
54-91-1   7634

$C_{10}H_{16}Br_2N_2O_2$
1,4-Bis(3-bromopropionyl)-piperazine. Amedel; pipobroman; NSC-25154; A-1803; A-8103. Antineoplastic agent. mp = 106-107°. *Abbott Labs.*

381   Verteporfin
129497-78-5

$C_{14}H_{22}N_2O \cdot HCl \cdot H_2O$
2-(Diethylamino)-N-(2,6-dimethyl-phenyl)acetamide hydrochloride
monohydrate.   Lignocaine
hydrochloride; Versicane; Lidesthesin;
Lignavet; Odontalg; Sedagul; Xylocard;
Xyloneural. Local anesthetic. *May &
Baker Ltd.;   Rhône-Poulenc   Rorer
Pharmaceuticals Inc.*

382   Vinblastine
865-21-4   10119

$C_{46}H_{58}N_4O_9$
Vincaleukoblastine.
vinblastine; VLB; 29060-LE; NSC-49842.
Antineoplastic agent. Antitumor alkaloid
isolated from *Vinca Rosea*. mp = 211-
216°; $[\alpha]_D^{26}$ = 42° (CHCl$_3$); practically
insoluble in H$_2$O, petroleum ether;
soluble in alcohols, Me$_2$CO, EtOAc,
CHCl$_3$. *Eli Lilly & Co.*

383   Vinblastine Sulfate
143-67-9   10119 205-606-0

$C_{46}H_{60}N_4O_{13}S$
Vincaleukoblastine sulfate.
vinblastine sulfate; 29060-LE; Velsar;
Belvan; Exal; Vincaleukoblastine sulfate
(1:1) (salt); VLB monosulfate; Velbe;
Velban; NSC-49842. Antineoplastic
agent. mp = 284-285°; $[\alpha]_D^{26}$ = -28° (c =
1.01 in MeOH). *Eli Lilly & Co.*

384   Vincamine
1617-90-9   10120 216-576-3

$C_{21}H_{26}N_2O_3$
(3α,14β,16α)-14,15-Dihydro-14-
hydroxyeburnamenine-14-carboxylic
acid methyl ester.
Angiopac;   Arteriovinca;   Devincan;
Equipur; Novicet; Ocu-vinc; Oxygeron;
Perval; Pervincamine; Pervone; Sostenil;
Tripervan;   NSC-91998;   Vincadar;
Vincafarm;   Vincafolina;   Vincafor;
Vincagil;   Vincalen;   Vincamidol;
Vincapront;   Vinvasaunier;   Vincimax;
Vinodrel Retard; Vraap. Antineoplastic
agent. Alkaloid isolated from *vinca
minor*. mp = 232-233°; $[\alpha]_D^{23}$ = 41°
(C$_5$H$_5$N); λ_m = 225, 278 nm (log ε 4.14,
3.61); LD$_{50}$ (mus orl) = 1000 mg/kg.

385   Vincristine Sulfate
2068-78-2   10124   218-190-0

$C_{46}H_{56}N_4O_{10}.H_2SO_4$
22-Oxo-vincaleukoblastinesulfate (1:1)
(salt) (9CI).
Kyocristine; Leurocristine sulfate; Lilly
37231; LCR; Oncovin; Onkovin;
Vincristine sulfate; Vincristine, sulfate;
Vincrisul; VCR sulfate; 37231; NSC-
67574. Antineoplastic agent. *Eli Lilly &*
Co.

386   Vindesine
53643-48-4   10125

$C_{43}H_{55}N_5O_7$
3-Carbamoyl-4-deacetyl-3-
de(methoxycarbonyl)vincaleukoblastine.
Compound 112531; desacetylvinblastine
amide; VDS; NSC-245467.
Antineoplastic agent. Synthetic
derivative of the alkaloid vinblastine. mp
= 230-232°; $[\alpha]_D^{25}$ = 39.4° (MeOH c = 1);
λ_m = 214, 266, 288, 296 nm (ε 53400,
17450, 13950, 12500 MeOH); pKa'
(H_2O) = 6.04, 7.67. *Eli Lilly & Co.*

387   Vindesine Sulfate
59917-39-4   10125

$C_{43}H_{57}N_5O_{11}S$
3-Carbamoyl-4-deacetyl-3-
de(methoxycarbonyl)vincaleukoblastine
sulfate.
Eldisine; LY-099094; NSC-245467.
Antineoplastic agent. mp > 250°; LD_{50}
(mus iv) = 6.3 mg/kg, 8.8 mg/kg, (rat iv) =
2.0 mg/kg. *Eli Lilly & Co.*

388   Vinepidine
68170-69-4

$C_{46}H_{56}N_4O_9$
(4'S)-4'-Deoxyleurocristine.
LY-119863. Antineoplastic agent. *Eli Lilly*
& Co.

389   Vinepidine Sulfate
83200-11-7
$C_{46}H_{58}N_4O_{13}S$
(4'S)-4'-Deoxyleurocristine sulfate.
Antineoplastic agent. *Eli Lilly & Co.*

390　Vinflunine
162652-95-1

$C_{45}H_{54}F_2N_4O_8$
20',20'-Difluoro-3',4'-dihydro-
vinorelbine.
A fluorinated Vinca alkaloid.
Antineoplastic agent.

391　Vinfosiltine
123286-00-0

$C_{51}H_{72}N_5O_{10}P$
[23(S)]-4-Deacetyl-3-
de(methoxycarbonyl)-3-[(2-methyl-1-
phosphonopropyl)carbamoyl]vincaleuko
blastine diethyl ether.
S-12363. Vinca alkaloid derivative.
Antineoplastic.

392　Vinglycinate
865-24-7

$C_{48}H_{63}N_5O_9$
4-Deacetylvincaleukoblastine 4-(N,N-
dimethylglycinate) (ester).
Antineoplastic agent. *Eli Lilly & Co.*

393　Vinglycinate Sulfate
7281-31-4
$C_{48}H_{63}N_5O_9 \cdot 1.5H_2SO_4$
4-Deacetylvincaleukoblastine 4-(N,N-
dimethylglycinate) (ester) sulfate (2:3)
salt.
Antineoplastic agent. *Eli Lilly & Co.*

394　Vinleucinol
81571-28-0

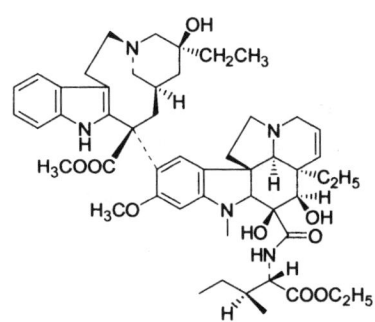

$C_{51}H_{69}N_5O_9$
[23(1S,2S)]-4-Deacetyl-3-[(1-carboxy-2-
methylbutyl)carbamoyl]-3-
de(methoxycarbonyl)vincaleukoblastine
ethyl ether.
VileE; vinblastine-isoleucinate. Vinca
alkaloid derivative. Antineoplastic.

395 Vinleurosine
23360-92-1

$C_{46}H_{56}N_4O_9$
Leurosine.
Leurosine; Lilly 32645; NSC-528004. Antineoplastic agent. Alkaloid isolated from Madagascar periwinkle. *Eli Lilly & Co.*

396 Vinleurosine Sulfate
1404-95-1
$C_{46}H_{58}N_4O_{13}S$
Leurosine sulfate.
Leurosine sulfate; Lilly 32645; NSC-528004. Antineoplastic agent. Sulfate salt of alkaloid isolated from Madagascar periwinkle. *Eli Lilly & Co.*

397 Vinorelbine
71486-22-1   10127

$C_{45}H_{54}N_4O_8$
3',4'-Didehydro-4'-deoxy-8'-norvincaleukoblastine.
Antineoplastic agent. $[\alpha]_D^{20} = 52.4°$ (CHCl$_3$ c = 0.3); λ_m = 215, 268, 282,293, 310 nm (ϵ 3700, 11000, 9500, 7600, 4400 EtOH). *Glaxo Wellcome Inc.*

398 Vinorelbine Tartrate
125317-39-7   10127
$C_{53}H_{66}N_4O_{20}$
3',4'-Didehydro-4'-deoxy-8'-norvincaleukoblastine L-(+)-tartrate. Navelbine. Antineoplastic agent. Soluble in H$_2$O, EtOH. *Glaxo Wellcome Inc.*

399 Vinrosidine
15228-71-4

$C_{46}H_{58}N_4O_9$
4'-Deoxy-3'-hydroxy vincaleucoblastine. Antineoplastic agent. Alkaloid isolated from Vinca rosea Linne. *Eli Lilly & Co.*

400 Vinrosidine Sulfate
18556-44-0

$C_{46}H_{58}N_4O_9 \cdot xH_2SO_4$
4'-Deoxy-3'-hydroxy vincaleucoblastine sulfate.
36781. Antineoplastic agent. Sulfate salt of alkaloid isolated from *Vinca rosea* Linne. *Eli Lilly & Co.*

401   Vintriptol
81600-06-8

$C_{56}H_{68}N_6O_9$
[23(S)]-4-Deacetyl-3-[(1-carboxy-2-indol-3-ylethyl)carbamoyl]-3-de(methoxycarbonyl)vincaleukoblastine diethyl ether.
Vinblastine tryptophan ester. Vinca alkaloid derivative; a tryptophan ester of vinblastine. Antineoplastic.

402   Vinzolidine Sulfate
67699-41-6

$C_{48}H_{60}ClN_5O_{13}S$
Methyl (3R,5S,7R,9S)-9-[3'-(2-chloro-ethyl)-6,7-didehydro-4β-hydroxy-16-methoxy-1-methyl-2',4'-dioxo-2β,3β,5α,12β,19α-spiro[aspidos-permidine-3,5'-oxazolidin]-15-yl]-5-ethyl-1,4,5,6,7,8,9,10-octahydro-5-hydroxy-2H-3,7-methanoazacyclo-undecino[5,4-b]indole-9-carboxylate-4'-acetate (ester) sulfate (1:1) (salt).
LY-104208. Antineoplastic agent. *Eli Lilly & Co.*

403   Vorozole
129731-10-8

$C_{16}H_{13}ClN_6$
(+)-(S)-6-(p-Chloro-α-1H-1,2,4-triazol-1-ylbenzyl)-1-methyl-1H-benzotriazole.
R-83842. Antineoplastic agent. *Janssen Pharmaceutical Inc.*

404   Zanosar
18883-66-4   8991   242-646-8

$C_8H_{15}N_3O_7$
2-deoxy-2-[[(Methylnitrosoamino)-carbonyl]amino]-D-glucose.
NSC-37917; NSC-85998; Streptozoticin; Streptozotocin, Pure; STZ; U-9889; Zanosar. Antineoplastic agent. mp = 115° (dec); soluble in H_2O, lower alcohols, ketones; λ_m = 228 nm (ε 6360); LD_{50} (mus ip) = 360 mg/kg. *Pharmacia & Upjohn, Inc.*

405   Zeniplatin
111490-36-9

$C_{11}H_{20}N_2O_6Pt$
cis-[2,2-Bis(aminomethyl)-1,3-propanediol](1,1-cyclobutane-dicarboxylato)platinum.
CL-286558. Antineoplastic agent.

406   Zinostatin
9014-02-2

Neocarzinostatin.
Antineoplastic agent. Polypeptide derived from *Streptomyces carzinostaticus* var. *Bristol-Myers Squibb Pharmaceutical Res. and Dev.*

407   Zinostatin Stimalamer
123760-07-6

Neocarzinostatin stimalamer.
Antineoplastic agent. Derivative of polypeptide derived from *Streptomyces carzinostaticus* var. *Bristol-Myers Squibb Pharmaceutical Res. and Dev.*

408   Zorubicin
54083-22-6   10326

$C_{34}H_{35}N_3O_{10}$
Benzoic acid hydrazide 3-hydrazone with daunorubicin.
Antineoplastic agent. *Rhône-Poulenc.*

409   Zorubicin Hydrochloride
36508-71-1   10326

$C_{34}H_{36}ClN_3O_{10}$
Benzoic acid hydrazide 3-hydrazone with daunorubicin monohydrochloride.
RP-22050 hydrochloride; NSC-164011.
Antineoplastic agent. $[\alpha]_D^{20}$= -50°; λ_m = 232.5, 253, 480, 495 nm (ε 40225, 35300, 10480, 10300 MeOH); LD_{50} (mus sc) = 13.66 mg/kg, (mus ip) = 4.42 mg/kg, (mus iv) = 8.50 mg/kg. *Rhône-Poulenc.*

Cytoprotectant Agents

410   Aceglutamide Aluminum
12607-92-0   25

$C_{35}H_{59}Al_3N_{10}O_{24}$
Pentakis (N²-acetlL-glutaminato)-terahydroxytrialuminum.
Glumal; KW-110. Anti-ulcerative. mp = 221° (dec); soluble in H_2O; practically insoluble in MeOH, EtOH, Me_2CO; LD_{50} (mmus orl) = 14.3 g/kg, (mmus ip) = 5.0 g/kg, (mmus iv) = 0.46 g/kg, (mrat orl) > 14.5 g/kg, (mrat ip) = 4.2 g/kg, (mrat iv) = 0.40 g/kg. *Kyowa Hakko Kogyo Co., Ltd.*

411   Acetoxolone
6277-14-1   76   228-475-1

$C_{32}H_{48}O_5$
(20β)-3β-(acetyloxy)-11-oxoolean-12-en-29-oic acid.
acetylglycyrrhetinic acid; glycyrrhetic acid acetate. Anti-ulcerative. Derivative of enoxolone; homolog of carbenoxolone mp = 322-325°; $[α]_D^{20}$ = 141°; insoluble in H_2O; soluble in most organic solvents; LD_{50} (mrat orl, ip) > 3000 mg/kg. *Dott. Inverni & Della Beffa.*

412   Acetoxolone Aluminum Salt
29728-34-5   76   249-815-5

$C_{96}H_{141}AlO_{15}$
(20β)-3β-(Acetyloxy)-11-oxoolean-12-en-29-oic acid aluminum salt.
Oriens. Anti-ulcerative. mp = 286-290°; $[α]_D^{20}$ = 126° ±2° (c = 1 $CHCl_3$); insoluble in H_2O; LD_{50} (mrat orl) > 3300 mg/kg. *Dott. Inverni & Della Beffa.*

413   Benexate Hydrochloride
78718-25-9   1065

$C_{23}H_{28}ClN_3O_4$
trans-2-[[[4-[[(Aminoiminomethyl)-amino]methyl]cyclohexyl]carbonyl]oxy] benzoic   acid   phenmethyl   ester monohydrochloride.
Anti-ulcerative. Synthetic protease inhibitor. mp = 83°. *Nippon Chemiphar.*

414   Carbenoxolone
5697-56-3   1839   227-174-2

$C_{34}H_{50}O_7$
3β-Hydroxy-11-oxoolean-12-en-30-oic acid hydrogen succinate.

Anti-ulcerative. mp = 291-294°; $[\alpha]_D^{20}$ = 128° (CHCl$_3$). *Biorex*.

415 Carbenoxolone Sodium
7421-40-1   1839   231-044-0

$C_{34}H_{48}Na_2O_7$
3β-Hydroxy-11-oxoolean-12-en-30-oic acid hydrogen succinate disodium salt.
Biogastrone; Bioplex; Bioral; Duogastrone; Neogel; Pyrogastrone; Sanodin; Ulcus-Tablinen; 18β-glycyrrhetic acid hydrogen succinate. Anti-ulcerative. A proprietary preparation of carbenoxolone sodium; a gastro-intestinal sedative. Anti-inflammatory gluccocorticoid related to enoxolone. soluble in H$_2$O; LD$_{50}$ (mmus ip) = 120 mg/kg, (mmus iv) = 198 mg/kg, (mrat orl) = 3200 mg/kg. *Biorex*.

416 Cetraxate
34675-84-8   2067

$C_{17}H_{23}NO_4$
p-Hydroxyhydrocinnamic acid trans-4-(aminomethyl)cyclohexanecarboxylate.
tramexamic acid p-(2-carboxyethyl)-phenyl ester; Anti-ulcerative. Derivative of tranexamic acid. mp = 200-280°. *Daiichi Seiyaku*.

417 Cetraxate Hydrochloride
27724-96-5   2067

$C_{17}H_{24}ClNO_4$
p-Hydroxyhydrocinnamic acid trans-4-(aminomethyl)cyclohexanecarboxylate hydrochloride.
DV-1006; Neuer. Anti-ulcerative. Derivative of tranexamic acid. mp = 238-240°. *Daiichi Seiyaku*.

418 Guaiazulene
489-84-9   4581   207-701-2

$C_{15}H_{18}$
1,4-Dimethyl-7-(1-methylethyl)azulene.
S-guaiazulene; AZ 8; AZ 8 Beris; Eucazulen; Kessazulen; Vaumigan. Anti-inflammatory and anti-ulcerative. Blue oil; bp$_{10}$ = 165-170°.

419 Irsogladine
57381-26-7   5113

$C_9H_7Cl_2N_5$
2,4-Diamino-6-(2,5-dichlorophenyl)-s-triazine.
dicloguamine. Anti-ulcerative. mp = 268-269°. *Nippon Shinyaku*.

420   Irsogladine Maleate
84504-69-8   5113

$C_{13}H_{11}Cl_2N_5O_4$
2,4-Diamino-6-(2,5-dichlorophenyl)-s-triazine maleate.
MN-1695; Gaslon. Anti-ulcerative. mp = 205° (dec); LD_{50} (mmus orl) = 6035 mg/kg, (mmus sc) = 2841 mg/kg, (mmus ip) = 775 mg/kg, (fmus orl) = 5697 mg/kg, (fmus sc) = 3216 mg/kg, (fmus ip) = 1006 mg/kg, (mrat orl) = 3898 mg/kg, (mrat sc) = 1600 mg/kg, (mrat ip) = 558 mg/kg, (frat orl) = 2917 mg/kg, (frat sc) = 1524 mg/kg, (frat ip) = 545 mg/kg. *Nippon Shinyaku.*

421   Nitecapone
116313-94-1

$C_{12}H_{11}NO_6$
3-(3,4-Dihydroxy-5-nitrobenzylidene)-2,4-pentanedione.
OR-462. Nitrocatechol-type catechol-O-methyltransferase inhibitor. Antioxidant; cytoprotectant.

422   Picoprazole
78090-11-6

$C_{17}H_{17}N_3O_3S$
Methyl 6-methyl-2-[[(3-methyl-2-pyridyl)methyl]sulfinyl]-5-benzimidazolecarboxylate.

H 149/94. A benzimidazole derivative that suppresses acid secretion through inhibition of (H+/K+)-ATPase. Antiulcerative; cyctoprotectant.

423   Plaunotol
64218-02-6   7692

$C_{20}H_{34}O_2$
(2Z,6E)-2-[(3E)-4,8-Dimethyl-3,7-nona-dienyl]-6-methyl-2,6-octadiene-1,8-diol.
CS-684; Kelnac. Anti-ulcerative. Soluble in organic solvents, insoluble in H_2O; LD_{50} (mmus orl) = 8800 µl/kg, (fmus orl) = 8100 µl/kg, (mrat orl) = 10900 µl/kg, (frat orl) = 11200 µl/kg. *Sankyo.*

424   Polaprezinc
107667-60-7   7712

$(C_9H_{12}N_4O_3Zn)_n$
[N-β-Alanyl-L-histidinato(2-)-N,N^N,O^α]-zinc.
zinc L-carnosine; Z-103; Promac. Anti-ulcerative. Has antioxidant and gastroprotective properties. Insoluble in H_2O; LD_{50} (mmus ip) = 220 mg/kg, (mmus sc) = 758 mg/kg, (mmus orl) = 1269 mg/kg, (fmus ip) = 165 mg/kg, (fmus sc) = 874 mg/kg, (fmus orl) = 1331 mg/kg, (mrat ip) = 405 mg/kg, (mrat sc) > 5000 mg/kg, (mrat orl) = 8441 mg/kg, (frat ip) = 422 mg/kg, (frat sc) > 5000 mg/kg, (frat orl) = 7375 mg/kg. *Hamari.*

425 Rebamipide
90098-04-7   8296

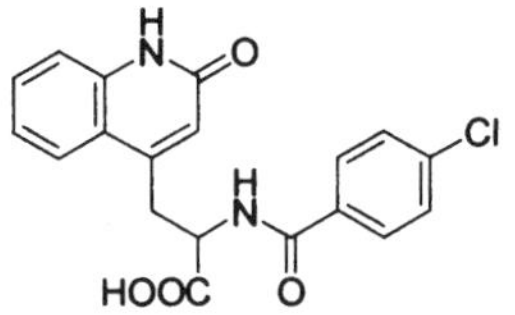

$C_{19}H_{15}CIN_2O_4$
(±)-α-(p-Chlorobenzamido)-1,2-dihydro-
2-oxo-4-quinolinepropionic acid.
OPC-12759; Mucosta; proamipide. Anti-
ulcerative. Gastric cytoprotectant. mp=
288-290° (dec). *Otsuka America
Pharmaceuticals, Inc.*

426 Sofalcone
64506-49-6   8850

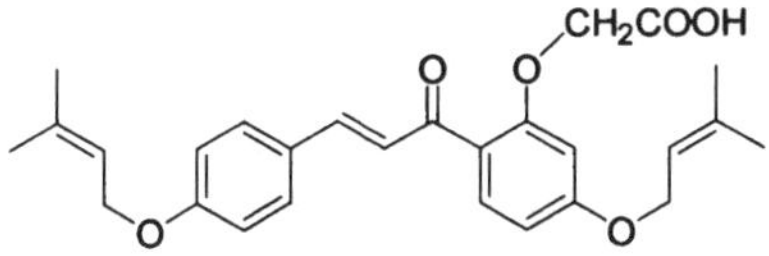

$C_{27}H_{30}O_6$
[5-[(3-Methyl-2-butenyl)oxy]-2-[p-[(3-
methyl-2-butenyl)oxy]cinnamoyl]-
phenoxy]acetic acid.
Su-88; Solon. Anti-ulcerative. mp = 143-
144°; LD_{50} (mus, rat orl) > 10 g/kg.
Taisho.

427 Spizofurone
72492-12-7   8918

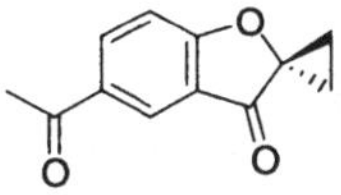

$C_{12}H_{10}O_3$
5-Acetylspiro[benzofuran-2(3H),1'-
cyclopropan]-3-one.
AG-629; Maon. Anti-ulcerative. mp =
102-104°, 106-107°. *Takeda.*

428 Sucralfate
54182-58-0   9049   259-018-4

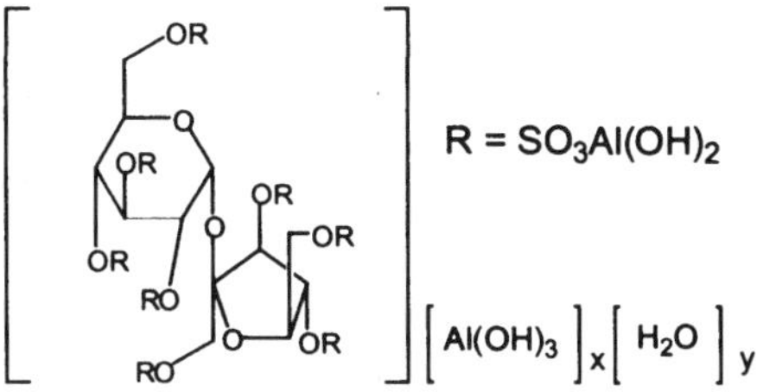

$R = SO_3Al(OH)_2$

$C_{12}H_mAl_{16}O_nS_8$
Sucrose octakis(hydrogen sulfate)
aluminum complex.
Carafate; Antepsin; Citogel; Hexagastron;
Keal; Succosa; Sucralfin; Sucrate; Sugast;
Sulcrate; Ulcar; Ulcerlmin; Ulcogant.
Gastrointestinal anti-ulcerative. Insoluble
in H_2O, EtOH; soluble in dilute HCl and
NaOH solutions. *Hoechst Marion
Roussel Inc.; Chugai Pharmaceutical Co.,
Ltd.*

429 Sulglicotide
54182-59-1
Sulfuric polyester of a glycopeptide
isolated from pig duodenum.
sulglycotide. A sulfoglycopeptide.
Antiulcerative; cytoprotectant.

430 Teprenone
6809-52-5   9296

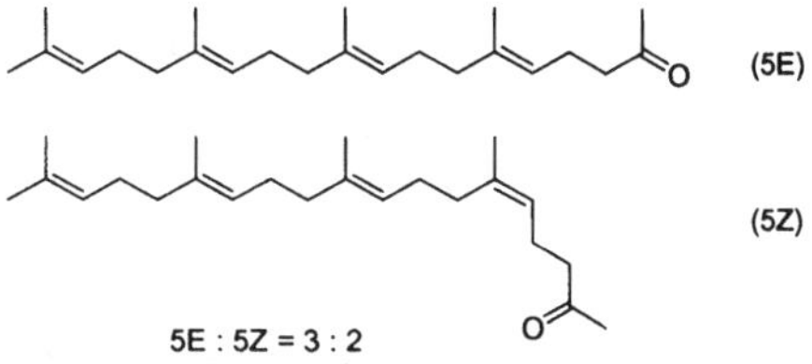

(5E)

(5Z)

5E : 5Z = 3 : 2

$C_{23}H_{38}O$
6,10,14,18-Tetramethyl-5,9,13,17-
nonadecatetraene-2-one; mixture of
(5E,9E,13E) and (5Z,9E,13E) isomers.
geranylgeranylacetone; GGA; E-0671;
E36U31; Selbex. Anti-ulcerative. $bp_{0.01}$=
155-160°; $d_4^{20.5}$= 0.9081.

431   Troxipide
99777-81-8   9921

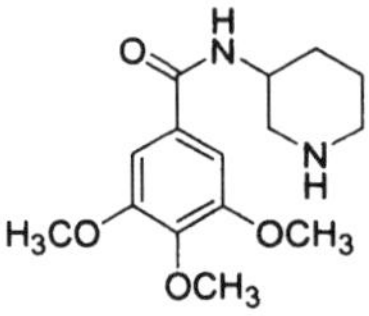

$C_{15}H_{22}N_2O_4$

(±)-(3,4,5-Trimethoxy-N-3-piperidyl-
benzamide.

KU-54; Aplace. Anti-ulcerative. mp=
179-185°; soluble in EtOH; LD_{50} (mrat
orl) = 500 mg/kg, (mrat sc) > 4150
mg/kg, (mrat ip) = 340 mg/kg, (frat orl) =
2100 mg/kg, (frat sc) > 4150 mg/kg, (frat
ip) = 340 mg/kg, (mmus orl) = 2200

mg/kg, (mmus sc) = 1600 mg/kg, (mmus
ip) = 300 mg/kg, (fmus orl) = 2000
mg/kg, (fmus sc) = 1550 mg/kg, (fmus ip)
= 305 mg/kg. *Kyorin*.

432   Zolimidine
1222-57-7   10320   214-947-4

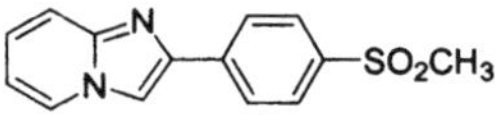

$C_{14}H_{12}N_2O_2S$

2-[4-(Methylsulfonyl)phenyl]imidazo-
[1.2-a]-pyridine.

zoliridine; Solimidin. Anti-ulcerative.
Non-cholinergic gastroprotective agent.
mp = 242-244°; LD_{50} (rat orl) = 3710
mg/kg; [hydrochloride]: LD_{50} (mus ip) =
800 mg/kg. *Selvi*.

PART II

INDEXES

INDEXES

1. CAS Registry Number Index

CAS Registry Number Index

CAS Registry Number Index

CAS Registry Number Index

CAS Registry Number Index

2. EINECS Number Index

EINECS Number Index

3. Name and Synonym Index

Name and Synonym Index

Name and Synonym Index

Name and Synonym Index

Name and Synonym Index

Name and Synonym Index

Name and Synonym Index

Name and Synonym Index

Name and Synonym Index

Name and Synonym Index

Name and Synonym Index

Name and Synonym Index

Name and Synonym Index

Name and Synonym Index

Name and Synonym Index

Name and Synonym Index

PART III

MANUFACTURERS AND SUPPLIERS DIRECTORY

MANUFACTURERS AND SUPPLIERS

3M Company
3M Center
St Paul, MN 55144
USA
Tel: +1 (612) 733-1110

3M Health Care
3M Center
St Paul, MN 55144
USA
Tel: +1 (612) 733-1110

3M Health Care Ltd
1 Morley Street
Loughborough,
Leics LE11 1EP
England
Tel: +44 (01509) 611611

3M Pharmaceuticals
3M Center 2751
St Paul, MN 55144-1000
USA
Tel: +1 (612) 733-0266
Fax: +1 (612) 737-2759

Abbott Laboratories
100 Abbott Park Rd
Abbott Park, IL 60064
USA
Tel: +1 (847) 937-6100
Fax: +1 (847) 937-1511

Abbott Laboratories Ltd
Abbott House
Moorbridge Rd
Maidenhead,
Berks SL6 8JG
England
Tel: +44 (01628) 773355

ABIC
Address Unknown

Adria Labs
Direct Inquiries to
Pharmacia & Upjohn

Advanced Magnetics, Inc
Corporate Headquarters
61 Mooney St
Cambridge, MA 02138
USA
Tel: +1 (617) 497-2070
Fax: +1 (617) 547-2445

**Agouron
Pharmaceuticals, Inc**
10350 North Torrey Pine Rd
La Jolla, CA 92037
USA
Tel: +1 (858) 622-3000

Ajinomoto Co, Inc
1-15-1, Kyobashi
Chuo-ku Tokyo 104
Japan
Tel: +81 (3) 5250-8111

Ajinomoto-Takara Corp
2-17-11, Kyobashi
Chuo-ku Tokyo 104
Japan
Tel: +81 (3) 3563-7589
Fax: +81 (3) 3535-3689

Aktieselskabet Pharmacia
Direct Inquiries to
Pharmacia & Upjohn

Akzo Chemie
Stationsplein 4
PO Box 247
NL-3800 Le Amersfort
The Netherlands

Akzo Nobel
Terhulpsesteenweg 166
Chee de la Hulpe 166
Brussels
Belgium
Tel: +32 (2) 663 5533

Albemarle Asano Corp
16th Floor
Fukoku Seimei Bldg
2-2, Uchisaiwaicho,
2-Chome
Chiyoda-ku, Tokyo 100
Japan
Tel: +81 (3) 5251-0791
Fax: +81 (3)3500-5623

**Albemarle Asia Pacific
Corp**
111 Somerset Road #13-03
Singapore 238164
Singapore
Tel: +65 732-6286
Fax: +65 737-4155

Albemarle Corp
451 Florida St
Baton Rouge, LA
70801-1785
USA
Tel: +1 (225) 388-7402
Fax: +1 (225) 388-7848

Albemarle SA
Parc Scientifique Einstein
Rue du Bosquet 9
B-1348 Louvain La Neuve Sud
Belgium
Tel: +32 (10) 48-1711
Fax: +32 (10) 48-1717

**Albright & Wilson Ameri-
cas, Inc**
4851 Lake Brook Dr
PO Box 4439
Glen Allen, VA 23060
USA
Tel: +1 (804) 968-6300
Fax: +1 (804) 968-6385

Albright & Wilson Ltd
PO Box 3
210-222 Hagley Rd
West Oldbury
W Midlands B68 ONN
England
Tel: +44 (0121) 429 4942
Fax: +44 (0121) 420 5151

Alcon Japan Ltd
Koraku Kokusai Bldg
1-5-3, Koraku, Bunkyo-ku
Tokyo 112
Japan
Tel: +81 (3) 3812-7881
Fax: +81 (3)3812-0188

Alcon Laboratories
PO Box 6600
6201 South Freeway
Fort Worth, TX 76115
USA
Tel: +1 (817) 293 0450

Alfa Wassermann SpA
Viale Sarca 223
20173 Milano
Italy
Tel: +39 (02) 64222-310

Allchem Industries
6010 NW First Place
Gainesville, FL 32607
USA
Tel: +1 (352) 378-9696
Fax: +1 (352) 338-0400

Allen & Hanbury
Direct Inquiries to Glaxo
Wellcome

Allergan Herbert
2525 DuPont Dr
Irvine, CA 92713
USA
Tel: +1 (714) 246-4500
Fax: +1 (714) 246-6987

Allergan, Inc
2525 Dupont Dr
PO Box 19534
Irvine, CA 92623-9534
USA
Tel: +1 (714) 246-4500
Fax: +1 (714) 246-6987

Alliance Pharm Corp
3040 Science Pk Dr
San Diego, CA 92121
USA
Tel: +1 (858) 410-5200
Fax: +1 (858) 410-5201

Alpha 1 Biomedicals, Inc
Two Democracy Center
6903 Rockledge Dr
Bethesda, MD
20817-1129
USA
Tel: +1 (301) 564-4400
Fax: +1 (301) 564-4424

Altana, Inc
60 Baylis Rd
Melville, NY 11747
USA
Tel: +1 (516) 454-7677
Fax: +1 (516) 454-0732

American Cyanamid
5 Garret Mountain Plaza
West Patterson, NJ 07470
USA
Tel: +1 (973) 357-3100

American Home Products
Five Giralda Farms
Madison, NJ 07940
USA
Tel: +1 (973) 660-5000
Fax: +1 (973) 660-5771

American Hospital Supply
20 Wiggins Ave
Bedford, MA 01730
USA
Tel: +1 (781) 275-1100

Amersham Corp
2636 South Clearbrook Dr
Arlington Heights, IL
60005
USA
Tel: +1 (847) 593-6300
Fax: +1 (847) 593-8075

Amersham International plc
Amersham Place
Little Chalfont
Amersham
Bucks HP7 9NA
England
Tel: +44 (01494) 544000

Amgen, Inc
Amgen Center
Thousand Oaks, CA
91320-1799
USA
Tel: +1 (805) 447-1000
Fax: +1 (805) 447-1010

**Amylin Pharmaceuticals,
Inc**
9373 Town Center Dr
San Diego, CA 92121
USA
Tel: +1 (858) 552-2200
Fax: +1 (858) 552-2212

Manufacturers and Suppliers Directory

Anaquest
Address Unknown

Angelini Francesco
Address Unknown

Angelini Group, Italy
Viale Amelia 70
00181 Rome
Italy
Tel: +39 (06) 78053-1
Fax: +39 (06) 78053-291

Angelini Pharmaceuticals, Inc
70 Grande Ave
River Edge, NJ 07661
USA
Tel: +1 (201) 489-4100

Anphar
Address Unknown

Anphar-Rolland
BP 203
91007 Evry Cedex
France
Tel: +33 (1) 64 97 20 30
Fax: +33 (1) 64 97 05 84

Antibiotice SA
1 Valea Lupului Street
Lasi 6600
Romania
Tel: +40 (32) 211010
Fax: +40 (32) 211020

Apothecon
Direct Inquiries to
Bristol-Myers Squibb Co

Apothekernes
Direct Inquiries to ASTRA
USA Inc

Arizona
1001 E Business 98
Panama City, FL 32401
USA
Tel: +1 (850) 785-6700
Fax: +1 (850) 785-2203

Armour Pharmaceuticals Co Ltd
St Leonards Road
Eastbourne
East Sussex BN21 3YG
England
Tel: +44 (01323) 410200

Asahi Chem Industry
Lyoner Str 44-48
D-60528 Frankfurt
Germany

Ascher, BF & Co
15501 W 109th St
PO Box 717
Shawnee Mission, KS 66201
USA
Tel: +1 (913) 888-1880

Asta Chemische Fabrik
Direct Inquiries to ASTA
Medica

Asta Medica AB
Kemistvagen 17
SE-18379 Taby
Sweden

Asta Medica AG
Weissmullerstr 45
D-60314 Frankfurt am Main
Germany
Tel: +49 69 400101
Fax: +49 69 40012740

ASTA Medica Inc
Continental Plaza, Tower 1
401 Hackensack Ave
Hackensack, NJ 07601
USA
Tel: +1 (201) 525-2680
Fax: +1 (201) 488-8595

ASTA Medica Ltd
168 Cowley Road
Cambridge CB4 0DL
England
Tel: +44 (01223) 423434
Fax: +44 (01223) 420943

Asta-Werke AG
Direct Inquiries to Asta
Medica

Astra Chemicals Ltd
Direct Inquiries to
AstraZeneca

Astra Draco AB
BO Box 34
Lund SE-221 00
Sweden
Tel: +46 (46) 336000

Astra Hässle AB
Karragatan 5
Molndal SE 431 83
Sweden
Tel: +46 (31) 7761000

Astra Pharmaceuticals Ltd
Home Park Estate
King's Langley,
Herts WD4 8DH
England
Tel: +44 (01923) 266191
Fax: +44 (01923) 260431

Astra USA, Inc
Direct Inquiries to Astra
Zeneca

AstraZeneca
1800 Concord Pike
PO Box 15437
Wilmington, DE 19850
USA
Tel: +1 (302) 886-3000
Fax: +1 (302) 886-2972

Athena Neurosciences, Inc
800 Gateway Blvd
S. San Francisco, CA 94080
USA
Tel: +1 (650) 877-0900
Fax: +1 (650) 877-8370

Atrix Laboratories
2579 Midpoint Dr
Fort Collins, CO
80525-4417
USA
Tel: +1 (970) 482-5868
Fax: +1 (970) 482-9735

Ayerst
Direct Inquiries to
Wyeth-Ayerst Laboratories

Ayrton Saunders plc
34 Hanover Street
Liverpool
Merseyside
England

Bacillofabrik Dr Bode & Co
Address Unknown

BASF Corp
3000 Continental Dr
Mt Olive, NJ 07828
USA
Tel: +1 (973) 426-2800
Fax: +1 (973) 426-2810

Basic Inc
Address Unknown

Battle Hayward & Bower Ltd
Crofton Drive
Allenby Rd Industrial Estate
Lincoln
Lincs LN3 4NP
England
Tel: +44 (01522) 529206

Bausch & Lomb Pharmaceuticals, Inc
One Bausch & Lomb Place
Rochester, NY 14604
USA
Tel: +1 (716) 338-6000

Bausch & Lomb Vision Care Division
1400 N Goodman St
Tampa, FL 33637
USA
Tel: +1 (813) 975-7700

Baxter Healthcare Systems
One Baxter Parkway
Deerfield, IL 60015
USA
Tel: +1 (847) 948-4731

Bayer AG
Werk Leverkusen
D-51368 Leverkusen
Germany
Tel: +49 214 301
Fax: +49 214 306 6328

Bayer Animal Health
12707 Shawnee Mission
Pk PO Box 390
Shawnee Mission, KS 66201
USA
Tel: +1 (913) 631-4800

Bayer Corp
Pharmaceutical Div
400 Morgan Lane
West Haven, CT 06516
USA
Tel: +1 (203) 937-2000

Bayer Corp, Pharmaceutical Div
400 Morgan Lane
West Haven, CT 06516
USA
Tel: +1 (203) 937-2000

BDH Laboratory Supplies
Broom Road
Parkstone
Poole
Dorset BH15 1TD
England
Tel: +44 (01202) 660444
Fax: +44 (01202) 666856

Becton Dickinson Microbiology Systems
1 Becton Dr
Franklin Lakes, NJ 07417
USA
Tel: +1 (201) 847-6800

Beecham Group plc
Four New Horizons Court
Harlequin Ave
Brentford
Middx TW8 9EP England
Tel: +44 (020) 8975 2000

Beecham Research Labs,
Direct Inquiries Beecham
Group plc

Beiersdorf AG
Aliothstr 40
CH-4142 Münchenstein 2
Switzerland
Tel: +41 (61) 415-6111
Fax: +41 (61) 415-6332

Beiersdorf AG
Unnastr 48
D020245 Hamburg
Germany
Tel: +49 40 49090
Fax: +49 40 49093434

Beiersdorf Inc
Wilton Corporate Center
187 Danbury Rd
Wilton, CT 06897
USA
Tel: +1 (203) 563-5800
Fax: +1 (203) 563-5895

Beiersdorf NV
Boulevard Industriel 30
B-1070 Bruxelles
Belgium
Tel: +32 (2) 526-5211
Fax: +32 (2) 526-5219

Beiersdorf Ltd
Yeomans Drive, Blakelands
Milton Keynes
Bucks MK14 5LS
England
Tel: +44 (01908) 211333
Fax: +44 (01908) 211555

Benz Research and Dev Corp
6447 Parkland Dr
PO Box 1839
Sarasota, FL 34230-1839
USA
Tel: +1 (941) 758-8256

Berk Pharmaceuticals Ltd
Brampton Road
Eastbourne
East Sussex BN22 9AG
England
Tel: +44 (01323) 501111

Berlex Laboratories, Inc
300 Fairfield Rd
Wayne, NJ 07470-7358
USA
Tel: +1 (973) 694-4100

Bilhuber
Address Unknown

BioCryst Pharmaceuticals, Inc
2190 Parkway Lake Dr
Birmingham, AL 35244
USA
Tel: +1 (205) 444-4600

Manufacturers and Suppliers Directory

BioDevelopment Corp
8180 Greensboro Dr
#1000
McLean, VA 22102
USA

Biofarma A/S
Naverland 22
DK-2600 Glostrup
Denmark
Tel: +45 4 327-0313

Biona A/S
DK-2860 Soeborg
Denmark
Tel: +45 3 969-2400
Fax: +45 3 969-2199

Bioproject
30, rue des
Francs-Bourgeois
75003 Paris
France
Tel: +33 (4) 42 71 71 16
Fax: +33 (4) 42 71 39 56

Biorex
PO Box 348
8201Vesprem-Szabadsapuszta
Hungary
Tel: +36 88-421-629
Fax: +36 88-429-237

Biorex Laboratories Ltd
2 Crossfield Chambers
Gladbeck Way
Enfield, Middx EN2 7HT
England
Tel: +44 (020) 8366 9301

Boehringer Ingelheim Ltd
Ellesfield Avenue
Bracknell
Berks RG12 8YS
England
Tel: +44 (01344) 424600

**Boehringer Ingelheim
Pharmaceuticals Inc**
900 Ridgebury Rd
Ridgefield Park, CT
06877-0103
USA
Tel: +1 (203) 798-9988

**Boehringer Ingelheim
GmbH**
Binger Str 173
D-55216 Ingelheim am
Rhein
Germany
Tel: +49 61 3277 5063
Fax: +49 61 3277 4225

**Boehringer Mannheim
GmbH**
Simpson Parkway
Kirton Campus
Livingston
West Lothian EH54 7BH
England
Tel: +44 (01589) 412512

Boots Company, The
1 Thane Road West
Nottingham
Oxon NG2 3AA
England
Tel: +44 (01602) 506111

Bottu
20, avenue Raymond Aron
92165 Antony Cedex
France
Tel: +33 140 91 61 23

Bracco Diagnostics, Inc
107 College Road E
Princeton, NJ 08540
USA

**Bristol-Myers Nutritional
Group**
725 E Main
Zeeland, MI 49464-0136
USA
Tel: +1 (616) 748-7100

Bristol-Myers Squibb Co
PO Box 4000
Princeton, NJ 08540
USA
Tel: +1 (609) 921-4000

**Bristol-Myers Squibb
Europe**
Le Grande Arche Nord
Paris La Défense Cedex
92044 Paris
France
Tel: +33 (1) 4090 6000
Fax: +33 (1) 4090 6100

**Bristol-Myers Squibb HIV
Products**
345 Park Ave
New York, NY
10154-0000
USA
Tel: +1 (212) 546-2856

**Bristol-Myers Squibb
Pharmaceutical Res and
Dev**
1 Squibb Drive
New Brunswick, NJ 08901
USA
Tel: +1 (201) 519-2000

**Bristol Myers Squibb
Pharmaceuticals Ltd**
Bristol Myers Squibb
House
141-149 Staines Rd
Hounslow
Middx TW3 3JA
England
Tel: +44 (020) 8572 7422

British Biotechnology Ltd
Watlington Rd
Oxford OX4 5LY
England
Tel: +44 (01865) 748747
Fax: +44 (01865) 781047

British Drug Houses
Direct Inquires to Merck

Brocades Ltd
Brocades House,
Pyrford Road
West Byfleet, Weybridge,
Surrey KT14 6RA
England
Tel: +44 (01932) 342291

**Brocades-Stheeman &
Pharmacia**
Direct Inquiries to
Pharmacia & Upjohn

**Broemmel
Pharmaceuticals**
3M Pharmaceuticals
3M Center, 275-3W01
St Paul, MN 55133-3275
USA

Buckeye Technologies
1001 Tillman St
PO Box 8407
Memphis, TN 38108
USA
Tel: +1 (901) 320-8100

Burroughs Wellcome
Direct Inquiries to
GlaxoWellcome

Byk Gulden Lomberg GmbH
Byk-Gulden-Str 2
Postfach 100310
7750 Konstanz
Germany
Tel: +49 7531 84 0
Fax: +49 7531 84 2474

C H Boehringer Sohn
Direct Inquiries to
Boehringer Ingelheim

CERM
Address Unknown

CM Industries
Erregierre Industria
Chimica SpA
Via Francesco Baracca, 57
24060 San Paolo D'Argon
(BG)
Italy
Tel: +39 (03) 595022

Cadus Pharmaceutical Corp
777 Old Saw Mill River Rd
Tarrytown, NY
10591-6705 USA
Tel: +1 (914) 345-3344
Fax: +1 (914) 345-3565

Calanda Stiftung
Address Unknown

California Research Co
Address Unknown

Callery Chemical
1420 Mars-Evans City Rd
Evans City, PA 16033
USA
Tel: +1 (412) 967-4141
Fax: +1 (412) 967-4140

Cambridge NeuroScience, Inc
One Kendall Square
Bldg 700
Cambridge, MA 02139
USA
Tel: +1 (617) 225-0600
Fax: +1 (617) 225-2741

Camillo-Corvi
Address Unknown

Carbide & Carbon Chem
Address Unknown

Carlo Erba Reagenti
Strada Rivoltana KM 6/7
20090 Rodano (Mi)
Italy
Tel: +39 (02) 9523 1
Fax: +39 (02) 95235904

Carrington Laboratories, Inc
2001 Walnut Hill Lane
Irving, TX 75038
USA
Tel: +1 (800) 527-5216
Fax: +1 (972) 518-1020

Carter-Wallace
PO Box 1001
Cranbury, NJ 08512
USA
Tel: +1 (609) 655-6000

Cassella AG
Hanauer Landstrasse 526
D-60386 Frankfurt
Germany
Tel: +49 (69) 4109 01
Fax: +49 (69) 4109 2650

CBD Corp
Address Unknown

Cell Therapeutics, Inc
201 Elliott Ave West, Ste
400
Seattle, WA 98119-4230
USA
Tel: +1 (206) 282-7100
Fax: +1 (206) 284-6206

Centeon LLC
1020 First Ave
King of Prussia, PA 19406
USA
Tel: +1 (610) 878-4000
Fax: +1 (610) 878-4009

Centocor, Inc
200 Great Valley Parkway
Malvern, PA 19355
USA
Tel: +1 (610) 651-6000
Fax: +1 (610) 889-4701

Centre d'Études l'Ind Pharm
Address Unknown

Cetus Corp
4560 Horton St
Emeryville, CA
94608-2997
USA
Tel: +1 (510) 653-5948

Chantal Pharmaceutical Corp
12121 Wilshire Blvd 1120
Los Angeles, CA
90025-1123
USA
Tel: +1 (310) 207-1950
Fax: +1 (310) 826-4214

Chantereau
Address Unknown

Chem Werke Albert
Address Unknown

Chem-Pharm Fabrik
Bahnhofstr 33-35 + 40
73033 Goeppingen
Germany
Tel: +49 7161 676-0
Fax: +49 7161 676-298

Chemex Pharmaceuticals
660 White Plains Rd
Ste 400
Tarrytown, NY 10591
USA
Tel: +1 (914) 332-8633

Chemiewerk Homburg
Address Unknown

Chemo Puro
Address Unknown

Chemoterapico
Address Unknown

Chimie et Atomistique
Address Unknown

Chinoin
1325 Budapest, Pf 110
H-1045 Budapest
Hungary
Tel: +36 (1) 169-0900
Fax: +36 (1) 169-0293

Chiron Corp
4560 Horton St
Emerville, CA 94608-2916
USA
Tel: +1 (510) 655-8730
Fax: +1 (510) 655-9910

Christiaens SA
Address Unknown

**Chugai Pharmaceutical
Co, Ltd**
Mulliner House, Flanders Rd
Turnham Green
London, W4 1NN
England
Tel: +44 (020) 8987-5600

CIBA plc
Direct Inquiries to Novartis

CIBA Vision AG
Grenzstr 10
CH-8180 Buelach
Switzerland
Tel: +41 (084) 880-8488
Fax: +41 (084) 880-8489

CIBA Vision Corp
11460 Johns Creek
Parkway
Duluth, GA 30097-1556
USA

CIBA Vision Ltd
Park West
Royal London Park
Flanders Rd, Hedge End
Southampton
Hants SO30 2LG
England
Tel: +44 (01489) 785580
Fax: +44 (01489) 786802

CIBA Vision Optics NL
4 Prinsenkade
NL-4811VB Breda
The Netherlands
Tel: +31 76-5245600
Fax: +31 76-5245620

Ciba-Geigy Corp
Direct Inquiries to Novartis

Cilag-Chemie Ltd
Saunderton
High Wycombe,
Bucks HP14 4HJ
England
Tel: +44 (01494) 563541

CIS-US, Inc
10 DeAngelo Dr
Bedford, MA 01730
USA
Tel: +1 (781) 275-7120
Fax: +1 (781) 275-2634

CK Witco (Europe) SA
7, rue du Pre-Bouvier
CH-1217 Meyrin
Switzerland
Tel: +41 (22) 989-2392

**CK Witco Asia Pacific Pte
Ltd**
12 Science Park Dr
118225 Singapore
Singapore
Tel: +65 770-5146

CK Witco Canada Ltd
565 Coronation Dr
West Hill, ON M1W 2K3
Canada
Tel: +1 (416) 284-6077

CK Witco Chemical Corp
One American Lane
Greenwich, CT
USA
Tel: +1 (203) 552-2747
Fax: +1 (203) 552-2882

CK Witco Chemical Ltd
Direct Inquires to Witco
(Europe) SA

Clin-Byk France
593, route de Boissise
77350 Le Mee-Sur-Seine
France
Tel: +33 (1) 64 41 22 22
Fax: +33 (1) 64 41 22 00

Clin-Byla France
593, route de Boissie
77350 Le Mee-Sur-Seine
France

Clin-Midy
9, rue du President Allende
94256 Gentilly Cedex
France
Tel: +33 (1) 40 73 40 73
Fax: +33 (1) 40 73 93 00

CNRS
16, rue Pierre et Marie
Curie
75005 Paris
France
Tel: +33 (1) 42 34 94 00
Fax: +33 (1) 43 26 87 23

Colgate-Palmolive
One Colgate Way
Canton, MA 02021
USA
Tel: +1 (908) 878-7500

**Consiglio Nazionale delle
Ricerche**
Via Tiburtina, 770
I-00159 Rome
Italy
Tel: +39 (06) 49932538
Fax: +39 (06) 49932440

Continental Pharma Inc
Address Unknown

Cook Imaging Corp
927 S Curry Pike B
Bloomington, IN 47403
USA
Tel: +1 (812) 333-0887
Fax: +1 (812) 332-3079

Cook-Waite Labs, Inc
Direct Inquires to Eastman
Kodak Co

Manufacturers and Suppliers Directory

Cooper Companies, Inc, The
10 Faraday
Irvine, CA 92618-1850
USA
Tel: +1 (949) 597-4700
Fax: +1 (949) 597-0662

Cooper Vision, Inc
200 Willow Brook Office Park
Fairport, NY 14450
USA

Corbiere
Address Unknown

Cortech, Inc
376 Main St
PO Box 74
Bedminster, NJ 07921
USA
Tel: +1 (908) 234-1881

Council of Scientific and Industrial Research, New Delhi
Address Unknown

Crinos
Piazza XX Settembre, 2
22079 Villa Guardia (C0)
Italy
Tel: +39 (031) 385111
Fax: +39 (031) 481784
wwcrinos-spacom

Crookes Healthcare Ltd
1 Thane Road West
Nottingham
NG2 3AA
England
Tel: +44 (01602) 506111

Cutter Laboratories
Direct Inquiries to Bayer Corp

Cypros Pharmaceutical Corp
2714 Loker Ave West
Carlsbad, CA 92008
USA
Tel: +1 (760) 929-9500
Fax: +1 (760) 929-8038

Cytogen Corp
600 College Rd
E Princeton, NJ 08540
USA
Tel: +1 (609) 987-8270
Fax: +1 (609) 951-9298

Daiichi Pharmaceutical Co Ltd
3-14-10, Nihonbashi
Chuo-ku, Tokyo 103
Japan
Tel: +81 (3) 3272-0611
Fax: +81 (3) 3272-8427

Daiichi Pharmaceutical Corp
11 Philips Parkway
Montvale, NJ 07645
USA
Tel: +1 (201) 573-7000

Daiichi Seiyaku
3-14-10, Nihonbashi
Chuo-ku, Tokyo 103
Japan
Tel: +81 (3) 3272-0611
Fax: +81 (3) 3272-8427

Dainippon Pharmaceutical
2-6-8, Dosho-machi
Chuo-ku, Osaka 541
Japan
Tel: +81 (6) 6203-5321
Fax: +81 (6) 6203-6581

Dautreville & Lebas
Address Unknown

Davis & Geck Medical Device Div
Direct Inquiries to
Wyeth-Ayerst Laboratories

DDSA Pharmaceuticals Ltd
Address Unknown

DeAngeli
Address Unknown

Degussa Ltd
Direct Inquires to
Degussa-Huls AG

Degussa-Huls AG
65 Challenger Rd
Ridgefield Park, NJ 07660
USA
Tel: +1 (201) 641-6100
Fax: +1 (201) 807-3183

Degussa-Huls AG
Headquarters
Weissfrauenstrasse 9
D-60311 Frankfurt am Main
Germany
Tel: +49 (69) 218-3618
Fax: +49 (69) 218-3849

Delagrange
1, avenue Pierre Brossolette
91380 Chilly Mazarin
France
Tel: +33 (1) 69 79 77 77
Fax: +33 (1) 69 79 75 75

Delandale Labs, Ltd
16, rue Henri Regnault
La Defense 6
92400 Courbevoie
France
Tel: +33 (1) 45 37 55 55
Fax: +33 (1) 49 00 02 93

Dermik Labs, Inc
Direct Inquires to
Rhône-Poulenc Rorer

Deutsche Hydrierwerke
Address Unknown

Dey Laboratories
2751 Napa Valley Corp Dr
Napa, CA 92558
USA
Tel: +1 (707) 224-3200
Fax: +1 (707) 224-3235

Dickinson, E E, Co
2 Enterprise Dr
Shelton, CT 06484-4666
USA
Tel: +1 (860) 388 3952

Diosynth BV
Vlijtseweg 130
PO Box 407
NL-7300 AK Apeldoorn
The Netherlands
Tel: +31 (55) 5286144
Fax: +31 (55) 5218808

Diosynth France SA
92821 Puteaux Cedex
France
Tel: +33 (1) 55 23 51 75

Dista Products Ltd
PO Box 25768
Alexandria, VA 22313
USA
Tel: +1 (800) 545-5979

Doak Pharmacal Co, Inc
67 Sylvester St
Westbury, NY 11590-4910
USA
Tel: +1 (516) 333-7222

Dome/Hollister-Stier
Direct Inquiries to Bayer
plc

Donau Pharm
Address Unknown

Dott Inverni & Della Beffa
Address Unknown

Dow Chemical USA
1803 Bldg
Midland, MI 48674
USA
Tel: +1 (517) 832-1000

Dumex Canada
104 Shorting Road
Toronto, ON M1S 3S4
Canada
Tel: +1 (416) 299-4003
Fax: +1 (416) 299-4912

Dumex USA
2250 Military Rd
Tonawanda, NY 14150
USA
Tel: +1 (800) 463-0106
Fax: +1 (716) 842-0707

DuPont Pharmaceutical Co
Experimental Sta 400/2413
PO Box 80400
Wilmington, DE 19880-0400
USA
Tel: +1 (302) 992-5000

DuPont Pharmaceuticals Ltd
Wedgwood Way
Stevenage
Herts SG1 4QN
England
Tel: +44 (01438) 842500

**DuPont-Merck
Pharmaceuticals**
Direct Inquiries to DuPont
Pharmaceuticals

**DuPont-Merck,
Radiopharmaceutical Div**
Direct Inquiries to DuPont
Pharmaceuticals

Dura Pharmaceuticals, Inc
7475 Lusk Blvd
San Diego, CA 92121
USA
Tel: +1 (619) 457-2553

Dynamit Nobel AG
Kaiserstr 1
Postfach 12 61
53839 Troisdorf
Germany
Tel: +49 (22) 41 89-0
Fax: +49 (22) 41 89-15 40

E Fougera & Co
60 Baylis Road
Melville, NY 11747
USA
Tel: +1 (516) 454-6996
Fax: +1 (516) 756-7017

E Geistlich Sohne
CH-6110 Wolhusen
Switzerland
Tel: + 41 710333

**E I Du Pont de Nemours
Inc**
1007 Market Street
Wilmington, DE 19898
USA
Tel: +1 (302) 774-7573

E Merck
Frankfurter Str 250
D-64293 Darmstadt
Germany
Tel: +49 61 51 72 0
Fax: +49 61 51 72 2000

ERASME
Address Unknown

Eastman Chemical Co
Fine Chemicals
PO Box 431
Kingsport, TN 37662
USA
Tel: +1 (423) 229-8124
Fax: +1 (423) 229-8133

Eastman Kodak
2/15/KO- Mailstop: 00539
343 State St
Rochester, NY 14650
USA
Tel: +1 (716) 724-4513
Fax: +1 (716) 724-0964

Eaton Labs
Address Unknown

ECR Pharmaceuticals
3981 Deep Rock Rd
PO Box 71600
Richmond, VA
23233-0141
USA
Tel: +1 (804) 527-1950

EGYT
Address Unknown

Eisai Co Ltd
4-6-10, Koishikawa
Bunkyo-ku, Tokyo 112-88
Japan
Tel: +81 (3) 3817-3700
Fax: +81 (3) 3811-3305

Eisai Corp of North Am
300 Frank W Burr Blvd
Teaneck, NJ 07666
USA
Tel: +1 (201) 692-9160

**Eisai Merrimack Valley
Laboratories, Inc**
100 Federal Street
Andover, MA 01810-0103
USA
Tel: +1 (978) 989-9911

Elan Pharmaceutical Research Corp
Lincoln House
Lincoln Place
Dublin 2
Ireland
Tel: +353 1 709-4000
Fax: +353 1 671-0920

Eli Lilly & Co
Lilly Corporate Center
Indianapolis, IN 46285
USA
Tel: +1 (317) 276-2000

Eli Lilly (Suisse) SA
PP Box 580
CH -1214 Venier/Geneva
Switzerland
Tel: +41 22-30-60-401

Eli Lilly Asia Pacific Pte Ltd
583 Orchard Road
#12-01/04
Forum
Singapore 238884
Tel: +65 732-2066

Eli Lilly Asia, Inc
Room 408, Man Po
International Center
660 Xin Hua Rd
Shanghai 200052
PR China
Tel: +86 21-6282-6008

Eli Lilly GmbH
Barichgasse 40-42
A-1030 Vienna
Austria
Tel: +43 (1) 711-780

Eli Lilly Group Ltd
Kingsclere Road
Basingstoke
Hants RG1 2XA
England
Tel: +44 (01256) 473241

Eli Lilly International Corporation
Lilly House
13 Hanover Square
London W1R OPA
England
Tel: +44 (020) 7409 4839

Eli Lilly Japan KK
Sannomiya Plaza Bldg
7-1-5, Isogami-dori
Chuo-ku, Kobe 651
Japan
Tel: +81 (8178) 242-9000

Elizabeth Arden
Direct Inquires to Eli Lilly

Elkins-Sinn
2 Esterbrook Lane
Cherry Hill, NJ
08002-4009
USA
Tel: +1 (610) 688-4400

EM Industries, Inc
Direct Inquiries to Merck
Hawthorne, NY 10532
USA
Tel: +1 (914) 592-4660
Fax: +1 (914) 592-9469

Endo Pharmaceuticals Inc
220 Lake Dr
Newark, DE 19702
USA
Tel: +1 (800) 462-3636
Fax: +1 (877) 329-3636

Enzon, Inc
40 Kingsbridge Rd
Piscataway, NJ 08854
USA
Tel: +1 (732) 980-4500
Fax: +1 (732) 980-5911

Enzypharm BV
Industrieweg 17
NL-3762 EG Soest
The Netherlands
Tel: +31 (35) 6030051
Fax: +31 (35) 6029962

Epoch Pharmaceuticals, Inc
1725 220th St SE, Ste 104
Bothell, WA 98021
USA
Tel: +1 (425) 485-8566

Eprova AG
Im Laternenacker 5
CH -8200 Schaffhausen
Switzerland
Tel: +41 (52) 630 7272
Fax: +41 (52) 630-7255

Esai Corp of North America
300 Frank W Burr Blvd
Teaneck, NJ 07666
USA
Tel: +1 (201) 692-9160

Esta Med Labs
Address Unknown

Esteve Group
Av Mare de Deu de
Montserrat, 221
8041 Barcelona
Spain
Tel: +34 93 446-6053
Fax: +34 93 433-0072

Esteve Group
Av Mare de Deu de
Montserrat, 12
8024 Barecelona
Spain
Tel: +34 93 284-6000
Fax: +34 93 284-6850

Ethicon, Inc
Route 22
Somerville, NJ 08876
USA
Tel: +1 (908) 218-0707

Ethyl Corp
330 South Fourth St
PO Box 2189
Richmond, VA 23218
USA
Tel: +1 (804) 788-5000
Fax: +1 (804) 788-5688

Evans Medical Ltd
Evans House
Regent Park, Kingston Rd
Leatherhead
Surrey KT22 7PQ
England
Tel: +44 (01372) 364000

F Hoffmann-LaRoche Ltd
CH-4070 Basel
Switzerland
Tel: +41 (61) 688 88 88
Fax: +41 (61) 688 27 75

Farbenfabriken Bayer AG
Address Unknown

Farmitalia Carlo Erba Ltd
Italia House
23 Grosvenor Rd
St Albans
Herts AL1 3AW
England
Tel: +44 (01727) 40041

Farmitalia, Societa Farmaceutici
Address Unknown

Farmos Group Ltd
PO Box 425
FIN-20101 Turku
Finland
Tel: +358 21 66 22 11

Ferlux-Chemie
24, Avenue d'Aubiere
63804 Cournon
d'Auvergne
France
Tel: +33 (4) 73 84 21 84
Fax: +33 (4) 73 84 21 80

Fermenta Animal Health Co
15th & Oak Street
PO Box 338
Elwood, KS 66024
USA

Ferrer
Address Unknown

Ferring Pharmaceuticals Inc
120 White Plains Rd
Tarrytown, NY 10591
USA
Tel: +1 (888) 337-7464

Ferrosan A/S
Corporate Headquarters
Sydmarken 5
DK-2860 Soeborg
Denmark
Tel: +45 3 969-2111
Fax: +45 3 969-6518

Ferrosan AB
Grynbodgatan 14
SE-21 33 Malmo
Sweden
Tel: +46 (40) 6607070
Fax: +46 (40) 6607089

Ferrosan AB
Kutojantie 11
(Vanvarsvagen)
FIN-02630 Espoo
Finland
Tel: +358 9 525 9050
Fax: +358 9 520 236

Ferrosan Ltd
69 Monmouth Street
London WC2H 9DG
England
Tel: +44 (020) 7240-2122
Fax: +44 (020) 7240-2188

Ferrosan Norge AS
Grini Naeringspark 1
1361 Osteras
Norway
Tel: +47 (6) 714-9505
Fax: +47 (6) 714-9530

Fidia Pharmaceuticals
Address Unknown

Fisons Pharmaceuticals Div
Rhône Poulenc Rorer
Mailstop 4C29, Box 5094
Collegeville, PA 19426-0998
USA
Tel: +1 (610) 454-8110

Fisons plc
Fison House
Princes St
Ipswich
Suffolk IP1 1QH
England
Tel: +44 (01473) 232525

Flint-Eaton
Address Unknown

FMC Corp, Pharm Div
1735 Market St
Philadelphia, PA 19103
USA
Tel: +1 (215) 299-6534
Fax: +1 (215) 299-6821

Forest Pharmaceuticals, Inc
13600 Shoreline Dr
St Louis, MO 63045
USA
Tel: +1 (800) 678-1605
Fax: +1 (314) 493-7450

Fujirebio Inc
2-7-1, Nishi-shinjuku
Shinjuku-ku
Tokyo 163-07
Japan
Tel: +81 (3) 3348-0691
Fax: +81 (3) 3342-6220

Fujisawa Pharmaceuticals Co, Ltd
3-4-7, Doso-machi
Chuo-ku, Osaka 541
Japan
Tel: +81 (6) 6202-1141
Fax: +81 (6) 6222-4988

Fujisawa Pharmaceuticals USA, Inc
3 Parkway North Center
Deerfield, IL 60015
USA
Tel: +1 (708) 317-0600

GAF
Direct Inquiries to Intl
Specialty Products, Inc

Galderma Canada, Inc
7300 Warden Ave, Ste 210
Markham, ON L3R 9Z6
Canada
Tel: +1 (905) 944-0717
Fax: +1 (905) 944-0790

Galderma Laboratories, Inc
3000 Alta Mesa Blvd
Ste 300
Fort Worth, TX 76133
USA
Tel: +1 (817) 263-2600
Fax: +1 (817) 263-2609

Gea A/S
Holger Danskes Vej 89
DK-2860 Frederiksberg
Denmark
Tel: +45 38 34 42 42
Fax: +45 38 34 11 23

Gedeon Richter Chem Works
Gyomroi ût 19-21
H-1103 Budapest
Hungary
Tel: +36 (1) 261 2199

Gelatin Products
Address Unknown

Manufacturers and Suppliers Directory

GenDerm
Medicis Pharmaceutical Corp
4343 E Camelback Rd
Phoenix, AZ 85018
USA
Tel: +1 (602) 808-8800
Fax: +1 (602) 808-0822

Genentech, Inc
1 DNA Way
So San Francisco, CA 94080
USA
Tel: +1 (650) 225-1000
Fax: +1 (650) 225-6000

General Aniline
Address Unknown

Genetics Institute, Inc
35 Cambridge Park Dr
Cambridge, MA 02140-2325
USA
Tel: +1 (617) 876-1170

Genta Inc
99 Hayden Ave, Ste 200
Lexington, MA
USA
Tel: +1 (781) 860-5150

Genzyme Corp
One Kendal Square
Cambridge, MA 02139
USA
Tel: +1 (617) 252-7500
Fax: +1 (617) 252-7600

Genzyme Ltd
37 Hollands Road
Haverhill
Suffolk CB9 8PU
England
Tel: +44 (01440) 703522

Gerda
6, rue Childebert
69002 Lyon
France
Tel: +33 (4) 72 77 69 19
Fax: +33 (4) 72 77 69 13

Gerot Pharmazeutika
Arnethgasse 3
A-1160 Vienna
Austria
Tel: +43 (1) 485 3505
Fax: +43 (1) 485 8932

Gilead Sciences, Inc
333 Lakeside Dr
Foster City, CA 94404
USA
Tel: +1 (650) 574-3000
Fax: +1 (650) 578-9264

Gist-Brocades International
PO 241068
8270 Red Oak Blvd, Ste 401
Charlotte, NC 28217
USA
Tel: +1 (704) 527-9000
Fax: +1 (704) 527-8844

Giuliani SpA
Via Palagi
2-20129 Milano
Italy
Tel: +39 (02) 20541
Fax: +39 (02) 29401341

Givaudan-Roure SA
55, rue de la Voie des Bancs
95100 Argenteuil
France
Tel: +33 (139) 98 15 15
Fax: +33 (139) 82 00 15

Glaxo Labs
Direct Inquiries to Glaxo
Wellcome

Glaxo Wellcome Inc
Five Moore Dr
PO Box 13398
Res Triangle Pk, NC 27709
USA
Tel: +1 (919) 248-2100
Fax: +1 (919) 248-7699

Glaxo Wellcome plc
Glaxo Wellcome House
Berkley Ave
Greenford
Middx UB6 0NN
England
Tel: +44 (0171) 4934060

Glenwood Inc
83 N Summit St
Tenafly, NJ 07670-0051
USA
Tel: +1 (201) 569-0050

Glidden Co
1900 Josey Lane
Carrolton, TX 75007
USA
Tel: +1 (214) 417-7400

Goodrich, BF, Co
Specialty Chemicals
9911 Brecksville Rd
Cleveland, OH 44141
USA
Tel: +1 (216) 447-6220
Fax: +1 (216) 447-6760

Goodrich, BF, Co, Europe
Specialty Chemicals
Rue de Verdun/straat 742
B-1130 Brussels
Belgium
Tel: +32 (2) 247-1911
Fax: +32 (2) 247-1990

Grace, WR & Co
Dewey & Almy Chemical Div
5225 Phillip Lee Dr
Altanta, GA 30336
USA
Tel: +1 (404) 691-8646

Greeff, RW & Co, LLC
777 West Putnam Ave
Greenwich, CT 06830
USA
Tel: +1 (203) 532-2900
Fax: +1 (203) 532-2980

Greenwich Pharmaceuticals, Inc
501 Office Center Drive
Ft Washington, PA 19034
USA

Grünenthal
Postfach 50 04 414
D-52088 Aachen
Germany
Fax: +49 0241 569-0

Grupo Farmaceutico Almirall SA
Maximo Aguirre 14
480940 Leioa
Spain
Tel: +34 94 4639000
Fax: +34 94 4646110

Gruppo Lepetit SpA
Via Murat 23
I-20159 Milano
Italy
Tel: +39 (2) 27 77 1

Guardian Laboratories
230 Marcus Blvd
PO Box 18050
Hauppauge, NY 11788
USA

Guilford Pharmaceuticals Inc
6611 Tributary St
Baltimore, MD 21224
USA
Tel: +1 (410) 631-6302
Fax: +1 (410) 631-6338

Hamari Chemicals Ltd
1-4-29, Shibajima
Higashiyodogawa-ku
Osaka 533
Japan
Tel: +81 (6) 6322-0191

Helopharm
Address Unknown

Herbert
Direct Inquiries to DuPont
Pharmaceuticals

Hercules Inc
1313 North Market St
Wilmington, DE 19894
USA
Tel: +1 (302) 594-5000
Fax: +1 (302) 594-5400

Hermes (GB) Ltd
7-9 Colville Road
London W3 8BL
England
Tel: +44 (020) 7259 5191

Heumann Pharma GmbH
Heideloffstr 18-28
90478 Neurnberg
Germany
Tel: +49 911 430 20
Fax: +49 911 430 24 15

Hexachemie
Address Unknown

Hexcel
Two Stamford Plaza
281 Tresser Blvd
Stamford, CT 06901
USA
Tel: +1 (203) 969-0666
Fax: +1 (203) 358-3977

Heyden Chemical
Address Unknown

Hindustan Antibiotics Ltd
Pune, Maharashtra
India

Hisamitsu Pharmaceutical Co Ltd
408 Tashirio Daikan-machi
Tosu-shi, Saga 841
Japan
Tel: +81 (942) 83 2101
Fax: +81 (942) 83 6119

Hoechst AG
D-65926 Frankfurt am Main
Germany
Tel: +49 69 305-2318
Fax: +49 69 305-83376

Hoechst AG (USA)
3 Park Ave
New York, NY 10016
USA
Tel: +1 (212) 251-8088
Fax: +1 (212) 251-8011

Hoechst Marion Roussel Inc
10236 Marion Park Dr
Kansas City, MO 64137-1405
USA
Tel: +1 (816) 966-4000
Fax: +1 (816) 966-3270

Hoechst Roussel Pharmaceuticals Inc
2110 East Galbraith
Cincinnati, OH 45215
USA
Tel: +1 (513) 948-9111

Hoechst Ltd
Hoechst House
Salisbury Rd
Hounslow
Middx TW4 6JH
England
Tel: +44 (020) 8570 7712

Hoffmann-LaRoche Inc
340 Kingsland St
Nutley, NJ 07110
USA
Tel: +1 (973) 235-5000

Hoffmann-LaRoche Ltd
CH-4070 Basel
Switzerland
Tel: +41 61 688 1111
Fax: +41 61 691 9391

Hokoriku
Address Unknown

Holding Ceresia
Address Unknown

Hommel GmbH
Postfach 1662
59336 Ludinghausen
Germany
Tel: +49 2591 23050
Fax: +49 02591 4413

Hooker Chemical
Direct Inquires to
Occidental Chemical Corp

Hovione
Sete Casas
2674-506 Loures
Portugal
Tel: +351 21 982 9000
Fax: +351 21 982 9388

Hybridon, Inc
155 Fortune Blvd
Milford, MA 01757
USA
Tel: +1 (508) 482-7500
Fax: +1 (508) 482-7510

Hyland Div, Baxter Healthcare Corp
One Baxter Parkway
Deerfield, IL 60015
USA
Tel: +1 (847) 948-4731

Hynson, Westcott & Dunning
Charles and Chase Sts
Baltimore, MD 21201
USA

IG Farben
Address Unknown

ISF
Address Unknown

Ibis Therapeutics
2292 Faraday Ave
Carlsbad, CA 92008
USA
Tel: +1 (760) 603-2700

ICI Americas Inc
Concord Plaza
Wilmington, DE 19897
USA
Tel: +1 (302) 886-3000
Fax: +2 (302) 886-2972

ICI Americas Inc
Concord Plaza
3411 Silverside Rd
Wilmington, DE 19850
USA
Tel: +1 (302) 887-3000

ICI Chemicals and Polymers Ltd
1900 Josey Lane
Carrolton, TX 75007
USA
Tel: +1 (214) 417-7400

ICN Pharmaceuticals, Inc
ICN Plaza
3300 Hyland Ave
Costa Mesa, CA 92626
USA
Tel: +1 (714) 545-0100
Fax: +1 (714) 556-0131

IDEC Pharmaceuticals Corp
11011 Torreyana Rd
San Diego, CA 92121
USA
Tel: +1 (619) 550-8500
Fax: +1 (618) 550-8750

Illumina
15817 Bernardo Center Dr
Ste 102
San Diego, CA
92127-2322
USA
Tel: +1 (619) 672-0419
Fax: +1 (619) 672-2325

Ilon Labs
Address Unknown

Immunetech Pharmaceuticals
Direct Inquiries to Dura
Pharmaceuticals

Immunex Corp
51 University St
Seattle, WA 98101
USA
Tel: +1 (206) 587-0430
Fax: +1 (206) 587-0606

Immunomedics, Inc
300 American Rd
Morris Plains, NJ 07950
USA
Tel: +1 (973) 605-8200
Fax: +1 (973) 605-8282

Imutec Pharma Inc
Direct Inquiries to Lorus
Therapeutics Inc

INDOFINE Chemical Co
PO Box 473
Somerville, NJ 08876
USA
Tel: +1 (908) 359-6778
Fax: +1 (908) 359-1179

Inex Pharmaceuticals Corp
1779 West 75th Avenue
V6P 6P2 Vancouver, BC
Canada
Tel: +1 (604) 264-9959

Innothera
7-9, avenue
Francois-Vincent Raspail
BP 12
94111 Arcueil Cedex
France
Tel: +33 (1) 46 15 18 00
Fax: +33 (1) 46 63 43 60

Inst Chemioter
Address Unknown

Inst Gentili SpA
Address Unknown

Inst Invest Desarr
Address Unknown

Inst Phys & Chem Res
Address Unknown

Interco Fribourg
Address Unknown

Interferon Sciences, Inc
783 Jersey Ave
New Brunswick, NJ
08901-3660
USA
Tel: +1 (732) 249-3250
Fax: +1 (732) 249-6895

International Specialty Products, Inc (ISP)
1361 Alps Rd
Wayne, NJ 07470
USA
Tel: +1 (201) 628-4000
Fax +1 (201) 628-4117

Interneuron Pharmaceuticals, Inc
1 Ledgemont Center
99 Hayden Ave, Ste 340
Lexington, MA 02173
USA
Tel: +1 (617) 861-8444
Fax: +1 (617) 861-3830

Investigacion Tecnica y Aplicada
Address Unknown

Iolab
2, Central Parc-Avenue
Sully Prudhomme
92298 Chatenay Malabry
Cedex
France
Tel: +33 (1) 43 50 80 80
Fax: +33 (1) 43 50 96

Irwin, Neissler
Address Unknown

Isis Pharmaceuticals, Inc
2292 Faraday Ave
Carlsbad, CA 92008
USA
Tel: +1 (619) 931-9200
Fax: +1 (619) 931-9639

ISP Van Dyk Inc
Address Unknown

Ist Biochim
Address Unknown
Ist De Angeli
Address Unknown

Italfarmaco SpA
Via dei Lavoratori, 54
20092 Cinisello Balsamo
(MI)
Italy
Tel: +39 (02) 64432301
Fax: +39 (02) 64432305

Janssen Pharmaceutical, Inc
1125 Trenton-Harbourton Rd
PO Box 200
Titusville, NJ 08560
USA
Tel: +1 (609) 730-2000

Janssen Pharmaceutical, Ltd
Grove
Wantage
Oxon OX12 0DQ
England
Tel: +44 (01235) 777333

Johnson & Johnson Medical Inc
One Johnson & Johnson Plaza
New Brunswick, NJ 08933
USA
Tel: +1 (732) 524-0400

Johnson & Johnson-Merck Consumer Pharmaceuticals
Camp Hill Rd
Fort Washington, PA 19034
USA

Jouveinal
1, rue des Moissons - BP 100
94265 Fresnes Cedex
France
Tel: +33 (1) 40 96 74 00
Fax: +33 (1) 46 68 16 44

Julian
Address Unknown

Juvantia Pharma Ltd
Tykistokatu 6A
FIN-20520 Turku
Finland
Tel: +358 2 333 7684
Fax: +358 2 333 7680

Kabi Pharmacia Diagnostics
800 Centiennial Ave
Piscataway, NJ 08540
USA

KabiVitrum AB
Direct Inquiries to
Pharmacia & Upjohn

Kaken Pharmaceutical Co, Ltd
1 Hinode
Urayasu-shi, Chiba 279
Japan
Tel: +81 (473) 90-6140
Fax: +81 (473) 90-6161

Kakenyaku Kako
Address Unknown

Kali-Chemie
Hans-Bockler-Allee 20
D-30173 Hannover
Germany
Tel: +49 511 8571
Fax: +49 511 282126

Kalle BV
Wetering 20
NL-6002 SM Weert
The Netherlands
Tel: +31 (495) 45 84 58
Fax: +31 (495) 45 87 44

Kanebo Cosmetics Ltd
Bone Lane
Newbury
Berks RG14 5TD
England
Tel: +44 (01635) 46362

Kanebo Pharmaceuticals Ltd
1-3-12, Motoakasaka
Minato-ku, Tokyo 107
Japan
Tel: +81 (3) 5411-3530
Fax: +81 (3) 5411-3568

Kefalas A/S
Address Unknown

Kendall McGaw Inc
2525 McGaw Ave
Irvine, CA 92614
USA
Tel: +1 (949) 660-2000

Key Pharmaceuticals
Direct Inquiries to
Schering-Plough

Keystone Chemurgic
Address Unknown

Kissei
Address Unknown

Klinge Pharma GmbH
Berg-am-Laim Str 129
81673 Munich
Germany
Tel: +49 69 4544-01
Fax: +49 69 4544-1329

Knoll Ltd
Fleming House
71 King St
Maidenhead
Berks SL6 1DU
England
Tel: +44 (01628) 776360

Knoll Pharmaceutical Co
3000 Continental Dr, North
Mt Olive, NJ 07828-1234
USA
Tel: +1 (800) 524-2474

Kobayashi Pharmaceutical Co, Ltd
2-7-16, Shoji-higashi
Ikuno-ku, Osaka 544
Japan
Tel: +81 (6) 6754-9522

Kowa Chemical Industries Co, Ltd
6-1-1, Heiwajima
Ohta-ku, Tokyo 143
Japan
Tel: +81 (3) 3767-3561
Fax: +81 (3) 3767-3917

Kreussler, Chemische-Fabrik
Rheingaustr 87-93
D-65203 Wiesbaden
Germany
Tel: +49 611 92710
Fax: +49 611 9271-111

KV Pharmaceutical
2503 S Hanley Rd
Saint Louis, MO
63144-2555
USA
Tel: +1 (314) 645-6600

Kyorin Pharmaceutical Co, Ltd
2-5, Kanda Surugadai
Chiyoda-ku, Tokyo 101
Japan
Tel: +81 (3) 3293-3411
Fax: +81 (3) 3293-6588

Kyowa Hakko Kogyo Co, Ltd
Ohtemachi Bldg
1-6-1 Ohte-machi
Chiyoda-ku, Tokyo 100
Japan
Tel: +81 (3) 3282-0007
Fax: +81 (3) 3284-1968

L Merckle GmbH
Graf-Arco-Str 3
89079 Ulm (Donau)
Germany
Tel: +49 731 402-01
Fax: +49 731 402-7832

Lab Albert Rolland
France Evry - Tour Lorraine
BP 203
91007 Evry Cedex
France
Tel: +33 (1) 64 97 20 30
Fax: +33 (1) 64 97 05 84

Lab Bouchara
66, rue Marjolin
92300 Levallois Perret
France
Tel: +33 (1) 45 19 10 00
Fax: +33 (1) 45 46 82 95

Lab Cassenne Marion
Tour Roussel-Hoechst
1, terrasse Bellini
92910 Paris La Defense
Cedex
France
Tel: +33 (1) 40 81 55 00
Fax: +33 (1) 40 81 40 82

Lab Dausse
Address Unknown

Lab Franc Chimiother
Address Unknown

Lab Houdé
Tour Roussel-Hoechst
1, terrasse Bellini
92910 Paris La Defense
Cedex
France
Tel: +33 (1) 40 81 42 00
Fax: +33 (1) 40 81 51 43

Lab Jacques Logeais
71, avenue du General de Gaulle
92137 Issy Les Moulineaux
Cedex
France
Tel: +33 (1) 46 45 21 99

Lab Laborec
Address Unknown

Lab Lafon, France
20, rue Charles Martigny
BP22
94701 Maisons Alfort
France
Tel: +33 (1) 49 81 81 00
Fax: +33 (1) 48 98 13 72

Lab Mauricio Villela SA
Address Unknown

Lab Meram
Avenue de la Liberation
77020 Melun Cedex
France
Tel: +33 (1) 64 87 20 50
Fax: +33 (1) 64 87 20 78

Lab Prod Biol Braglia
Address Unknown

Lab ProTer
Address Unknown

Labaz (Labs)
1, rue de la Viegre
33003 Bordeaux Cedex
France
Tel: +33 (56) 90 91 93

Labaz SA
9, rue du President Allende
94258 Gentilly Cedex
France
Tel: +33 (1) 40 73 63 00
Fax: +33 (1) 40 73 48 57

Laboratoire UPSA
128, rue Danton BP 325
92506 Rueil Malmaison
Cedex
France
Tel: +33 (1) 47 16 87 72
Fax: +33 (1) 47 16 87 78

Laboratoires Biocodex
19, rue Barbes
92126 Montrouge Cedex
France
Tel: +33 (1) 46 56 67 89
Fax: +33 (1) 40 92 17 61

Laboratorio Bago, SA
Address Unknown

Labs Fher SA
Address Unknown

Labs Franca Inc
Address Unknown

Labs OM
Address Unknown

Labs Sapos
Address Unknown

Lakeside BioTechnology
Address Unknown

Langley Smith Ltd
Address Unknown

Lark, SpA
Address Unknown

Laroche-Navarron
Address Unknown

Lederle Labs
Direct Inquiries to
Wyeth-Ayerst

Lee Laboratories
1475 Athens Highway
Grayson, GA 30221
USA
Tel: +1 (770) 972-4450
Fax: +1 (770) 979-9570

Lemmon Co
Direct Inquiries to Teva
Pharmaceuticals

Lentia
Address Unknown

Leo AB
55 Industriparken
Ballerup
DK-2750 Copenhagen
Denmark
Tel: +45 44 923 800
Fax: +45 44 943 040

Lever Brothers
Direct Inquiries to Unilever

Licencia Budapest
Address Unknown

Lion Dentrifice
Address Unknown

**Lipha Pharmaceuticals,
Inc**
1114 Ave of the Americas
41st Floor
New York, NY 10036
USA
Tel: +1 (212) 398-4602
Fax: +1 (212) 398-5021

Lipha Pharmaceuticals Ltd
Harrier House
High St, Yiewsley
West Drayton
Middx UB7 7QG
England
Tel: +44 (01895) 452200
Fax: +44 (01895) 420605

Lloyd, Hamol Ltd
Direct Inquiries to Reckitt
& Colman

Lombart Lenses Ltd, Inc
1215 Boissevain Ave
PO Box 1693
Norfolk, VA 23501
USA
Tel: +1 (757) 625-7866

Lorus Therapeutics, Inc
7100 Woodbine Ave
Ste 215
Markham ON L3R 5J2
Canada
Tel: +1 (905) 305-1100
Fax: +1 (905) 305-1584

Lovens Komiske Fabrik AS
Ramstadsletta 15
1322 Hovik
Norway
Tel: +47 (67) 12 30 03
Fax: +47 (67) 12 30 33

Lundbeck
37, ave Pierre 1er de
Serbie
75008 Paris
France
Tel: +33 (1) 53 67 42 00

Lundbeck GmbH & Co
Address Unknown

Lusofarmico
Address Unknown

Madan
Address Unknown

**Maggioni Farmaceutici
SpA**
Address Unknown

Mallinckrodt, Inc
7733 Forsyth Blvd
St Louis, MO 63105-1820
USA
Tel: +1 (314) 654-2000
Fax: +1 (314) 654-6510

Maltbie Chem
Address Unknown

Marion Merrell Dow Inc
Direct Inquires to Hoechst
Marion Roussel Inc

**Mar-Pha Soc Etud Exploit
Marques**
Address Unknown

Martin Dennis
Address Unknown

Maro Seiyaku
Address Unknown

Matieres Colorantes
255, rue de Paris
93100 Montreuil
France
Tel: +33 (1) 42 87 29 45
Fax: +33 (1) 42 87 10 39

Mauvernay
Address Unknown

May & Baker Ltd
Address Unknown

**McNeil Consumer
Products Co**
7050 Camp Hill Rd
Fort Washington, PA
19034
USA
Tel: +1 (215) 233 7000

McNeil Pharmaceutical
McKean and Welsh Rds
PO Box 13886
Spring House, PA 19477
USA

Mead Johnson Labs
Direct Inquiries to Bristol-
Myers Squibb Co

Mead Johnson Nutritionals
Direct Inquiries to Bristol-
Myers Squibb Co

Medco Research Inc
85 T Alexander Dr
PO Box 13886
Res Triangle Pk, NC 27709
USA
Tel: +1 (919) 549-8117
Fax: +1 (919) 549-7515

**Medical Market
Specialties, Inc**
Address Unknown

**Medicis Pharmaceutical
Corp**
4343 E Camelback Rd
Phoenix, AZ 85018
USA
Tel: +1 (602) 808-8800
Fax: +1 (602) 808-0822

**Mediolanum Farmaceutici
SpA**
Via SG Cottolengo, 15
20143 Milan
Italy
Tel: +39 (02) 8912-2232
Fax: + 39 (02) 8913-2375

Medi-Physics, Inc
2320 W Peoria Ave
Ste B-140-A
Phoenix, AZ 85029
USA
Tel: +1 (602) 371-8021

Medi-Physics, Inc
1341 Gene Autry Way
Anaheim, CA 92805
USA
Tel: +1 (714) 634-9633

**Meiji Milk Products Co,
Ltd**
2-3-6, Kyobashi
Chuo-ku, Tokyo 104
Japan
Tel: +81 (3) 3281-6118
Fax: +81 (3) 3281-4717

Meiji Seika Kaisha, Ltd
2-4-16, Kyobashi
Chuo-ku, Tokyo 104
Japan
Tel: +81 (3) 3272-6511
Fax: +81 (3) 3271-5792

**Menley & James
Laboratories, Inc**
100 Tournament Dr
Horsham, PA 19044
USA
Tel: +1 (215) 441-6500
Fax: +1 (215) 441-6576

Merck & Co Inc
One Merck Dr
PO Box 100
Whitehouse Sta, NJ 08889
USA
Tel: +1 (908) 423-1000
Fax: +1 (908) 594-4662

Merck KGaA
Frankfurter Str 250
D-64293 Darmstadt
Germany
Tel: +49 61 51-72-0
Fax: +49 61 51-72-2000

Merck Ltd
Merck House
Poole
Dorset BH15 1TD
England
Tel: +44 (01202) 669700

**Merck Pharmaceuticals
Ltd**
Harrier House
High St
West Drayton
Middx UB7 7QG
England
Tel: +44 (01895) 452200
Fax: +44 (01895) 420605

**Merck Sharpe & Dohme
Research Labs**
Hillsborough Rd
Three Bridges, NJ 08887
USA
Tel: +1 (908) 369-4900

**Merrell Dow
Pharmaceuticals Inc**
PO Box 9627
Kansas City, MO 64134
USA

Merrell Pharmaceuticals
Address Unknown

Microbiochem Res Found
Address Unknown

Miles Inc
One Mellon Center
500 Grant St
Pittsburgh, PA
15219-2502
USA
Tel: +1 (412) 394-5500
Fax: +1 (412) 394-5579

Mission Pharmacal Co
1325 East Durango Blvd
San Antonio, TX
78210-1771
USA
Tel: +1 (210) 553-7118

Mitsubishi Chemical Corp
Mitsubishi Bldg
5-2 Marunouchi 2-chome
Chiyoda-ku, Tokyo 100
Japan
Tel: +81 (3) 3283-6254
Fax: +81 (3) 3283-6287

Mitsubishi Kasei
Address Unknown

**Mitsui Pharmaceuticals,
Inc**
3-12-2, Nihonbashi
Chuo-ku, Tokyo 103
Japan
Tel: +81 (3) 3274-4711
Fax: +81 (3) 3281-4670

Mitsui Toatsu
Address Unknown

Mizzy
Address Unknown

Mobay
Direct Inquiries to
Monsanto

Mondi
Address Unknown

Monsanto Co
800 North Lindbergh Blvd
St Louis, MO 63167
USA
Tel: +1 (314) 694-1000

Mundipharma AG
Mundipharma Str 6
65549 Limburg (Lahn)
Germany

Muro Pharmaceuticals, Inc
890 East St
Tewksbury, MA
01876-1496
USA
Tel: +1 (978) 851-5981
Fax: +1 (978) 851-7346

N Am Philips
Address Unknown

NV Nederlandsche Comb Chem Ind
Address Unknown

NV Amsterdamsche Chininefabriek
Address Unknown

NV Philips
Address Unknown

National Cancer Institute
Bethesda, MD 20892

National Drug Co
Address Unknown

National Foundation for Cancer Research
Address Unknown

National Research Dev Corp
Address Unknown

Natterman
Address Unknown

Naugatuck
Address Unknown

Newport
Address Unknown

Nicholas Labs Ltd
Address Unknown

Nihon Nohyaku Co, Ltd
Eitaro Bldg
1-2-5 Nihonbashi
Chuo-ku, Tokyo 103
Japan
Tel: +81 (3) 3278-0461
Fax: +81 (3) 3281-5462

Nippon Chemiphar
2-2-3, Iwamoto-cho
Chiyoda-ku, Tokyo 101
Japan
Tel: +81 (3) 3863-1211
Fax: +81 (3) 3864-5940

Nippon Kayaku Co, Ltd
Tokyo Fujimi Bldg
1-11-2 Fujimi
Chiyoda-ku, Tokyo 102
Japan
Tel: +81 (3) 3237-5111
Fax: +81 (3) 3237-5091

Nippon Shinyaku, Japan
Hachijo Sagaru, Nishiohji
Minami-ku, Kyoto 601
Japan
Tel: +81 (75) 321-9105
Fax: +81 (75) 321-0400

Nissan Kenzai Co, Ltd
C/O Nissan Chemical
Industries, Toyama Factory
635, Sakakura,
Fuchu-machi
Nei-gun, Toyama 939-27
Japan
Tel: +81 (764) 65-6300
Fax: +81 (764) 65-6303

Nisshin Denka KK
2-2-1, Ohama
Sakata-shi, Yamagata 998
Japan
Tel: +81 (0234) 33-2121

Nisshin Kasei Co, Ltd
11-5, Senju Kawara-machi
Adachi-ku, Tokyo 120
Japan
Tel: +81 (3) 3888-1181
Fax: +81 (3) 3870-2121

Nopco
Address Unknown

Nordmark
Address Unknown

Norton, HN
Gemini House
Flex Meadows
Harlow
Essex CM19 5TJ
England
Tel: +44 (01279) 426666

Norwich
Direct Inquiries to Procter & Gamble

Norwich Eaton
Direct Inquiries to Procter & Gamble

Novartis Pharmaceuticals, Corp
59 Route 10
East Hanover, NJ
07936-1011
USA
Tel: +1 (908) 503-7500

Novo Nordisk Biotech, Inc
1445 Drew Ave
Davis, CA 95616
USA

Novo Nordisk Pharmaceuticals Inc
100 Overlook Center #2
Princeton, NJ 08540-7814
USA
Tel: +1 (609) 987-5800

Novocol Chem
Address Unknown

Novopharm Biotech, Inc
147 Hamelin Street
Winnipeg, MB R3T 3Z1
Canada
Tel: +1 (204) 478-1023
Fax: +1 (204) 452-7721

Occidental Chemical Corp
Occidental Tower
5005 LBJ Freeway
Dallas, TX 75244
USA
Tel: +1 (972) 404 3800

Oclassen Pharmaceuticals Inc
100 Pelican Way
San Rafael, CA 94901
USA
Tel: +1 (415) 258-4500
Fax: +1 (415) 258-4550

Octel Chemicals Ltd
PO Box 17, Oil Sites Road
Ellesmere Port
South Wirral L65 4HF
England
Tel: +44 (0151) 3553611

Manufacturers and Suppliers Directory

Oesterreiche Stickstoffwerke
Address Unknown

Ohio State University
Address Unknown

Olin Mathieson
Address Unknown

Olin Research Ctr
350 Knotter Dr
PO Box 586
Cheshire, CT 06410
USA
Tel: +1 (203) 271-4316
Fax: +1 (203) 271-4060

Omnium Chim
Address Unknown

O'Neal, Jones & Feldman Pharmaceuticals
Address Unknown

Ono Pharmaceutical
2-1-5, Dosho-machi
Chuo-ku, Osaka 541
Japan
Tel: +81 (6) 6222-5551
Fax: +81 (6) 6222-5706

Optacryl, Inc
2890 S Tejon St
Englewood, CO
80110-0120
USA
Tel: +1 (303) 789-0933

Optech, Inc
6341 Troy Circle
Englewood, CO
80111-0641
USA
Tel: +1 (303) 708-1390

Orgamol, SA
Address Unknown

Organon Inc
375 Mount Pleasant Ave
West Orange, NJ 07052
USA
Tel: +1 (201) 325-4500

Organon Laboratories Ltd
Science Park
Milton Rd
Cambridge CB4 4FL
England
Tel: +44 (01223) 423445

Orion Pharma
Orionintie 1
PO Box 65
FIN-02101 Espoo
Finland
Tel: +358 9 4291
Fax: +358 9 4293815

Orsymonde
Address Unknown

Ortho Biotech Inc
PO Box 670
700 US Highway 202
South
Raritan, NJ 08869-0670
USA
Tel: +1 (908) 704-5000

Ortho Diagnostic Systems Inc
US Route 202
Raritan, NJ 08869
USA
Tel: +1 (908) 218-8000

Ortho Pharmaceutical Corp
Route 202 South
Raritan, NJ 08869
USA
Tel: +1 (908) 704-1500
Fax: +1 (908) 526-4997

OSI Pharmaceuticals
106 Charles Lindbergh Blvd
Uniondale, NY
11553-3649
USA
Tel: +1 (516) 222-0023
Fax: +1 (516) 222-0114

OSSW
Address Unknown

Otsuka America Pharmaceutical
2440 Research Blvd Ste 500
Rockville, MD 20850
USA
Tel: +1 (301) 990-0030

Otsuka Pharmaceuticals Co Ltd
2-9, Kanda Tsukasa-cho
Chiyoda-ku
Tokyo 101-8535
Japan
Tel: +81 (3) 3292-0021

OXIS International, Inc
6040 North Cutter Circle
Ste 317
Portland, OR 97217
USA
Tel: +1 (503) 283-3911
Fax: +1 (503) 283-4058

Paines & Byme Ltd
Address Unknown

Paragon Vision Sciences
947 Elm Avenue
Mesa, AZ 85204
USA
Tel: +1 (480) 892 7602

Parke Davis & Co Ltd
Lambert Court
Chestnut Ave
Eastleigh Hamps SO5 3ZQ
England
Tel: +44 (01703) 620500

Parke-Davis
2800 Plymouth Rd
Ann Arbor, MI 48105
USA
Tel: +1 (734) 622-7000
Fax: +1 (734) 622-5229

Patchem, AG
Address Unknown

PCAS
Address Unknown

Penederm Inc
320 Lakeside Dr, Ste A
FosterCity, CA 94404
USA
Tel: +1 (415) 358-0100
Fax: +1 (415) 358-0101

Penick
Address Unknown

Penta Mfg
PO Box 1448
Fairfield, NJ 07007
USA
Tel: +1 (201) 740-2300
Fax: +1 (201) 740-1839

Pentapharm
Engelgasse 109
CH-4002 Basel
Switzerland
Tel: +41 (61) 706-9848
Fax: +41 (61) 319-9619

PerImmune, Inc
1330 Piccard Dr
Rockville, MD
20850-4396
USA
Tel: +1 (301) 258-5200

Permeable Technologies, Inc
712 Ginesi Dr
Morganville, NJ 07751
USA

Person & Covey, Inc
616 Allen Ave
Glendale, CA 91201-0201
USA
Tel: +1 (818) 240-1030

Perstorp AB
SE-28 4 80 Perstorp
Sweden
Tel: +46 (0) 435 3800
Fax: +46 (0) 435 3810

Pfalz & Bauer
172 E Aurora St
Waterbury, CT 06708
USA
Tel: +1 (203) 574-0075
Fax: +1 (203) 574-3181

Pfanstiehl Laboratories Inc
1219 Glen Rock Ave
Waukegan, IL 60085
USA
Tel: +1 (847) 623-0370
Fax: +1 (847) 623-9173

Pfizer Group Ltd
PO Box 2
Ramsgate Rd
Sandwich
Kent CT13 9NJ
England
Tel: +44 (01304) 616161

Pfizer Inc
Central Research
Eastern Point Rd
Groton, CT 06340
USA
Tel: +1 (860) 441-4100

Pfizer International
235 E 42nd St
New York, NY
10017-5755
USA

Pfleger (Dr R Pfleger)
96045 Bamberg
Germany
Tel: +49 951 60430
Fax: +49 951 604329

Pharm Res Products
Address Unknown

Pharmachemie
Swensweg 5
PO Box 552
2003 RN Haarlem
The Netherlands
Tel: +31 23 524 77 90
Fax: +31 23 514 77 74

Pharmacia
Direct Inquiries to
Pharmacia & Upjohn

Pharmacia & Upjohn
95 Corporate Dr
Bridgewater, NJ
08807-1265
USA
Tel: +1 (908) 306-4400
Fax: +1 (908) 306-4433

Pharmacia & Upjohn AB
Lindhagensgatan 133
SE-112 87 Stockholm
Sweden
Tel: +46 (08) 695 8000
Fax: +46 (08) 618 8607

Pharmacia & Upjohn, Inc
301 Henrietta St
Kalamazoo, MI 49001
USA
Tel: +1 (616) 323-4000
Fax: +1 (616) 323-4077

Pharmacia Hepar Inc
150 Industrial Dr
Franklin, OH 45005
USA
Tel: +1 (513) 746-3603

Pharmos Corp
Two Innovation Dr
Alachua, FL 32615
USA
Tel: +1 (904) 462-1210
Fax: +1 (904) 762-5401

Philips-Duphar BV
Address Unknown

Phillips
Specialty Chemicals
874 Adams Bldg
Bartlesville, OK 74004
USA
Tel: +1 (918) 661-9092
Fax: +1 (918) 661-8379

Pierre Fabre
5, ave Napoleon III - BP
497
74164 St Julien en
Genevois Cedex
France
Tel: +33 (4) 50 35 35 55
Fax: +33 (4) 50 35 35 90

Pierre Fabre
45, place Abel-Gance
92654 Boulogne Cedex
France
Tel: +33 (1) 49 10 80 00
Fax: +33 (5) 61 39 15 98

Pierrel SpA
Address Unknown

Pilkington Barnes Hind
810 Kifer Rd
Sunnyvale, CA 94086
USA
Tel: +1 (858) 614-7600

Pineapple Research Inst
Address Unknown

Pitman Moore Europe Ltd
Breakspear Road South
Harefield
Uxbridge
Middx UB9 6LS
England
Tel: +44 (01895) 626000

Pitman-Moore, Inc
1201 Douglas Ave
Kansas City, KS
66103-0140
USA
Tel: +1 (913) 321-1070

Polaroid
Address Unknown

Polfa
Address Unknown

Polichimica SpA
Address Unknown

Poythress
Address Unknown

Pratt Pharmaceuticals
Pfizer Inc
235 E 42nd St
New York, NY
10017-5755
USA

**Procter & Gamble
Pharmaceuticals, Inc**
11810 East Miami River Rd
Ross, OH 45061
USA
Tel: +1 (513) 983-1100

ProCyte Corp
12040 115th Ave NE
Ste 210
Kirkland, WA 98034-6900
USA
Tel: +1 (206) 820-4548
Fax: +1 (206) 820-4111

Promonta
Direct Inquiries to
Lundbeck GmbH

Provesan SA
Address Unknown

Purdue Pharma LP
100 Connecticut Ave
Norwalk, CT 06856
USA
Tel: +1 (203) 853-0123
Fax: +1 (203) 838-1576

Quimicobiol
Address Unknown

Quinoderm Ltd
Address Unknown

**RW Johnson Pharmaceuti-
cal Research Institute**
Route 202 South
PO Box 300
Raritan, NJ 08869-0602
USA
Tel: +1 (908) 704-4000

Raschig GmbH
Ludwigshafen
Germany

Ravensberg
Address Unknown

Ravizza
Address Unknown

Recherche et Ind Therap
Address Unknown

Reckitt & Colman Europe
One Burlington Lane
London W4 2RW
England
Tel: +44 (0181) 994-6464
Fax: +44 (0181) 944-8940

Reckitt & Colman Inc
1655 Valley Rd
Wayne, NJ 07470
USA
Tel: +1 (020) 8633 3600
Fax: +1 (020) 8633 3633

Recordati Corp
110 Commerce Dr
Allendale, NJ 07401
USA
Tel: +1 (212) 236-3669
Fax: +1 (212) 236-9404

**Recordati Industria
Chimica E Pharmaceutica
SpA**
Via M Civitali, 1
1-20148 Milano
Italy
Tel: +39 (02) 487 87536
Fax: +39 (02) 487 05223

Reed & Carnrick
65 Horse Hill Rd
Cedar Knolls, NJ 07927
USA
Tel: +1 (973) 267-2670

Refarmed
Address Unknown

Res Inst Pharm Chem
Address Unknown

Research Corp
Address Unknown

Resfar SRL
Address Unknown

Rexall Sundown, Inc
6111 Broken Sound
Parkway
Boca Raton, FL 33487
USA
Tel: +1 (561) 241-9400
Fax: +1 (561) 995-0197

Rhinepreussen AG
Address Unknown

Rhône-Poulenc
Direct Inquiries to
Rhône-Poulenc Rorer

Rhône-Poulenc Rorer
20, avenue Raymond Aron
92165 Antony Cedex
France
Tel: +33 (1) 55 71 71 71

Rhône-Poulenc Rorer Holdings Ltd
St Leonards House
52 St Leonard Rd
Eastbourne
East Sussex BN21 3YG
England
Tel: +44 (01323) 721422

Rhône-Poulenc Rorer Pharmaceuticals Inc
PO Box 1200
Collegeville, PA
19426-0107
USA

Richardson-Merrell
Direct Inquiries to Hoechst
Marion Roussel

Richardson-Vicks Inc
Direct Inquiries to Hoechst
Marion Roussel

Riedel de Haen (Chinosolfabrik)
Wunstorfer Str 40
30926 Seeize
Germany
Tel: +49 5137 999258
Fax: +49 5137 999674

Riker Labs
Direct Inquiries to 3M
Pharmaceuticals

Robert et Carriere
Address Unknown

Roberts Pharmaceutical Corp
4 Industrial Way West
Eatontown, NJ 07724
USA
Tel: +1 (732) 676-1200
Fax: +1 (732) 676-1300

Roche Laboratories
340 Kingsland St
Nutley, NJ 07110-1199
USA
Tel: +1 (973) 235-5000

Roche Products Ltd
40 Broadwater Road
Welwyn Garden City
Herts AL7 3AY
England
Tel: +44 (01707) 328128

Roche Puerto Rico
Direct Inquires to ICN
Pharmaceuticals

Roerig Div, Pfizer Pharmaceuticals
235 E 42nd St
New York, NY
10017-2399
USA

Rohm and Haas Co
100 Independence Mall W
Philadelphia, PA
19106-2399
USA
Tel: +1 (215) 785-8000

Rorer
Direct Inquiries to
Rhône-Poulenc Rorer

Ross Products
US Highway 29 North
PO Drawer 479
Altavista, VA 24517
USA
Tel: +1 (804) 369-3100

Roswell Park Memorial Inst
Buffalo, NY 14203
USA
Tel: +1 (716) 845-2300

Rotta Pharm
6, rue Casimir-Delavigne
75006 Paris
France
Tel: +33 (1) 44 07 12 44

Roussel Laboratories Ltd
Broadwater Park
North Orbital Rd, Denham
Uxbridge
Middx UB9 5HP
England
Tel: +44 (01895) 834343

Roussel-UCLAF
Direct Inquiries to Hoechst
Marion Roussel

Rowa Ltd
Newtown
Bantry, Cork
Ireland
Tel: +353 (027) 50077

Rowa-Wagner
Frankenforster Str 77
51427 Bergisch Gladbach
Germany
Tel: +49 2204 61081
Fax: +49 2204 61084

RW Johnson Pharmaceutical Research Institute, The
920 Route 202
PO Box 300
Raritan, NJ 08869-0602
USA
Tel: +1 (908) 704-4000

Rybar Labs Ltd
Address Unknown

Rystan Co, Inc
PO Box 214
Little Falls, NJ 07420-0214
USA
Tel: +1 (973) 256-3737

SIFA
Address Unknown

Salix Pharmaceuticals, Inc
3600 W Bayshore Rd
Ste 205
Palo Alto, CA 94303
USA
Tel: +1 (650) 856-1550

San NopCo Ltd
1-5-9, Nihonbashi
Hon-cho
Chuo-ku, Tokyo 103
Japan
Tel: +81 (3) 3279-3030
Fax: +81 (3) 3246-0550

Sandoz Pharmaceuticals Corp
Direct Inquires to Novartis
Pharmaceuticals

Sankyo Co, Ltd
3-5-1, Nihonbashi
Hon-cho
Chuo-ku, Tokyo 103
Japan
Tel: +81 (3) 5255-7111
Fax: +81 (3) 5255-7035

Sanofi Winthrop
301 Oxford Valley Rd
Morrisville, PA
19067-7706
USA
Tel: +1 (215) 321-7560

Sanofi Winthrop France
9, rue du President Allende
94258 Gentilly Cedex
France
Tel: +33 (1) 41 24 60 00
Fax: +33 (1) 41 24 63 00

**Santen Pharmaceutical
Co, Ltd**
3-9-19, Shimoshinjo
Higashiyodogawa-ku
Osaka 533
Japan
Tel: +81 (6) 6321-7045
Fax: +81 (6) 6325-8209

Savage Laboratories
60 Baylis Rd
Melville, NY 11747
USA
Tel: +1 (516) 454-7677
Fax: +1 (516) 454-0732

**Schein Pharmaceutical,
Inc**
620 N 51st Ave
Phoenix, AZ 85043-4705
USA
Tel: +1 (602) 278-1400
Fax: +1 (602) 447-3385

Schenley
Address Unknown

Schering AG
Muellerstr 170-178
D-13342 Berlin
Germany
Tel: +49 30 4681 111
Fax: +49 30 4681 5305

Schering Health Care Ltd
The Brow, Burgess Hill
West Sussex RH15 9BS
England
Tel: +44 (01444) 232323

**Schering-Plough
HealthCare Products**
110 Allen Road
Liberty Corner, NJ 07938
USA
Tel: +1 (908) 604-1640

Schering Plough Ltd
Chiswick Avenue, Field
Road Industrial Estate
Mildenhall
Bury St Edmunds
Suffolk IP28 7AX
England
Tel: +44 (01638) 716321

**Schering-Plough
Pharmaceuticals**
2015 Galloping Hill Rd
Kenilworth, NJ
07033-0530 USA
Tel: +1 (908) 298-4000

Schevico
Address Unknown

Schiapparelli
Direct Inquiries to Alfa
Wassermann

**Schwartz's
Essencefabriken**
Address Unknown

**Schwarz
Arztnelmittelfabrik**
Address Unknown

**Schwarz Pharma Kremers
Urban Co**
6140 Est Executive Dr
Mequon, WI 53092
USA

Schwarz Pharma Ltd
Schwarz House
East St
Chesham
Bucks HP5 1DG England
Tel: +44 (01494) 772071

Sci Union et Cie, France
Address Unknown

**SciClone Pharmaceuticals,
Inc**
901 Mariners Island Blvd
San Mateo, CA
94404-1593
USA
Tel: +1 (415) 358-3456
Fax: +1 (415) 358-3469

Scios Nova Inc
820 W Maude Ave
Sunnyvale, CA 94086
USA
Tel: +1 (408) 481-9177
Fax: +1 (408) 481-9188

**Scotia Pharmaceuticals,
Ltd**
Address Unknown

SCS Pharmaceuticals
Address Unknown

Searle Ltd
PO Box 53
Lane End Rd
High Wycombe
Bucks HP12 4HL
England
Tel: +44 (01494) 521124
Fax: +44 (01494) 447872

Searle, GD & Co
5200 Old Orchard Rd
Skokie, IL 60077
USA
Tel: +1 (847) 982-7000
Fax: +1 (847) 470-1480

Seceph
Address Unknown

Selvi
Address Unknown

Serono Laboratories, Inc
100 Longwater Circle
Norwell, MA 02061-0163
USA
Tel: +1 (781) 982-9000

Serono Laboratories Ltd
99 Bridge Road East
Welwyn Garden City
Herts AL7 1BG
England
Tel: +44 (01707) 331972

Shell
One Shell Plaza
Houston, TX 77252-2463
USA
Tel: +1 (713) 241-6161
Fax: +1 (713) 241-4043

Shionogi & Co, Ltd
3-1-8, Dosho-machi
Chuo-ku, Osaka 541
Japan
Tel: +81 (6) 6202-2161
Fax: +81 (6) 6229-9596

Siegfried AG
Address Unknown

**Sigma-Tau
Pharmaceuticals, Inc**
800 South Frederick Ave
Ste 300
Gaithersburg, MD 20877
USA
Tel: +1 (301) 948-1041
Fax: +1 (301) 948-3194

Sigma-Tau SpA
Industrie famaceutiche
riunite
Viale Shakespeare, 47
00144 Rome
Italy
Tel: +39 (6) 592-6443

Simes SpA
Address Unknown

Smith, T&H
Address Unknown

**SmithKline Beecham
Animal Health**
Direct Inquiries to Pfizer,
Inc

**SmithKline Beecham
Pharmaceuticals**
One Franklin Place
Philadelphia, PA 19102
USA
Tel: +1 (215) 751-3415
Fax: +1 (215) 751-7655

**Snow Brand Milk Products
Co, Ltd**
44 Montgomery St
San Francisco, CA 94104
USA
Tel: +1 (415) 677-0914

**Soc Belge Azote Prod
Chim Marly**
Address Unknown

Soc Belge des Labs Labaz
Address Unknown

**Soc Chim des Usines du
Rhône**
Address Unknown

Soc Chim Org Biol
Address Unknown

**Soc Etudes Sci Ind L'Île de
France**
Address Unknown

Soc Farmaceutici Italia
Address Unknown

**Soc Franc Recherches
Biochim**
Address Unknown

Soc Ind Fabric Antiboit
Address Unknown

Soc Italo-Brit L Manetti
Address Unknown

**Soc Italo-Brit L Manetti-H
Roberts**
Address Unknown

**Societa Prodiotti
Antibiotici, Italy**
Address Unknown

Societe Belge de l'azote
Address Unknown

Societe Berri-Balzac
Address Unknown

Sogeras
Address Unknown

Sola/Barnes-Hind
Direct Inquiries to Allergan
Inc

Solvay America, Inc
3333 Richmond Ave
Houston, TX 77098-3009
USA
Tel: +1 (713) 525-6000
Fax: +1 (713) 525-7887

Solvay Animal Health, Inc
1201 Northland Dr
Mendota Heights, MN
55120
USA
Tel: +1 (651) 681-3880
Fax: +1 (651) 681-9425

Solvay Deutschland GmbH
Hans-Bockler-Allee 20
D-30173 Hannover
Germany
Tel: +49 511-85-70
Fax: +49 511-28-21-26

**Solvay Duphar
Laboratories Ltd**
Duphar House, Gaters Hill
West End, Southampton,
Hamps SO3 3JD
England

**Solvay Pharmaceuticals
SA**
33, rue du Prince Albert
B-1050 Brussels
Belgium
Tel: +32 (2) 509 6111
Fax: +32 (2) 509 6304

**Solvay Pharmaceuticals,
Inc**
901 Sawyer Rd
Marietta, GA 30062
USA
Tel: +1 (770) 578-9000

Solvay Holding Co Ltd
Grovelands Business
Centre
Boundary Way
GB Hemel Hempstead
Herts HP2 7TE
England
Tel: +44 (01442) 236555
Fax: +44 (01442) 238770

Somerset Pharmaceuticals Inc
5215 W Laurel St
Tampa, FL 33607-0172
USA
Tel: +1 (813) 288-0040

Sonus Pharmaceuticals, Inc
22026 20th Ave SE
Bothell, WA 98021-4405
USA
Tel: +1 (206) 487-9500

SPA
Address Unknown

Sphinx Pharmaceutical Corp
20 T W Alexander Dr
Res Triangle PK, NC 27709
USA
Tel: +1 (919) 314-4000
Fax: +1 (919) 314-4350

SPOFA
Husinecka IIa
130 00 Praha 3
Czech Republic
Tel: +42 (2) 6278502
Fax: +42 (2) 6278320

Spojene
Direct Inquires to SPOFA

Squibb, ER & Sons
Direct Inquiries to
Bristol-Myers Squibb Co

Standard Oil Co, Indiana
Division of AMOCO Oil
Hc 331 Box S
Bremen, IN 46506
USA
Tel: +1 (219) 546-4342

Stauffer Chemical Co
Address Unknown

Stem Corporation
Woodrolfe Road
Tollesbury
Essex CM9 8SJ
England
Tel: +44 (01621) 868685
Fax: +44 (01621) 868445

Sterling Health USA
Direct Inquiries to Sanofi
Winthrop

Sterling Research Labs
Direct Inquiries to Sanofi
Winthrop

Sterling Winthrop, Inc
Direct Inquiries to Sanofi
Winthrop

Stiefel France
ZI du Petit Nantere
15, rue des Grands Pres
92007 Nanterre Cedex
France
Tel: +33 (1) 46 49 80 50
Fax: +33 (1) 47 82 99 72

Stiefel Laboratories, Inc
255 Alhambra Circle
Coral Gables, FL 33134
USA
Tel: +1 (305) 443-3800
Fax: +1 (305) 443-3467

Stokely-Van Camp
Oakland, CA 94601
USA
Tel: +1 (510) 261-3672

Stuart
Direct Inquiries to
AstraZeneca

Sumitomo Pharmaceuticals Co, Ltd
2-2-8, Dosho-machi
Chuo-ku, Osaka 541
Japan
Tel: +81 (6) 6229-5775
Fax: +81 (6) 6233-2399

Sun Pharmaceuticals Corp
1345 Pine Ave
Orlando, FL 32824-7942
USA
Tel: +1 (407) 859-3162

SunPharm Corp
4651 Salisbury Rd Ste 205
Jacksonville, FL 32256
USA
Tel: +1 (904) 296-3320

Suntory Ltd
2-1-40, Dojimahama
Kita-ku, Osaka 530
Japan
Tel: +81 (6) 6346-1131
Fax: +81 (6) 6345-1169

Synaptic Pharmaceutical Corp
215 College Rd
Paramus, NJ 07652
USA
Tel: +1 (201) 261-1331
Fax: +1 (201) 261-0623

Synergen, Inc
1885 33rd St
Boulder, CO 80301-2505
USA
Tel: +1 (303) 938-6200
Fax: +1 (303) 441-5535

Syntex International, Ltd
Direct Inquiries to Hoffman
LaRoche

Syntex Labs Inc
Boulder, CO
USA

Syntex Pharmaceuticalsl, Ltd
Syntex House
St Ives Rd
Maidenhead
Berks SL6 1RD
England
Tel: +44 (01628) 33191

Synthelabo Pharmacie
Lindberghstr 1
82178 Puchheim
Germany
Tel: +49 89 89017-0
Fax: +49 89 89017-299

Taiho
1-27, Kanda Nishiki-cho
Chiyoda-ku, Tokyo 101
Japan
Tel: +81 (3) 3294-4527
Fax: +81 (3) 3233-4318

Taisho
3-24-1, Takata
Toshima-ku, Tokyo 171
Japan
Tel: +81 (3) 3985-1111
Fax: +81 (3) 3982-9701

**Takeda Chemical
Industries, Ltd**
4-1-1, Dosho-machi
Chuo-ku, Osaka 541
Japan
Tel: +81 (6) 6204-2111
Fax: +81 (6) 6204-2880

**Tanabe Research
Laboratories, USA, Inc**
4540 Towne Centre Ct
San Diego, CA 92121
USA
Tel: +1 (619) 558-9211

Tanabe Seiyaku
Address Unknown

TAP Pharmaceuticals, Inc
Bannockburn Lake Office
Plaza
2355 Waukegan Rd
Deerfield, IL 60015
USA
Tel: +1 (847) 236-2270

TCI America
9211 North Harborgate St
Portland, OR 97203
USA
Tel: +1 (800) 423-8616
Fax: +1 (503) 283-1987

TechAmerica
Address Unknown

Teijin Ltd
Teijin Bldg
1-6-7, Minami-honmachi
Chuo-ku, Osaka 541
Japan
Tel: +81 (6) 6268-2132
Fax: +81 (6) 6266-1481

**Teikoku Hormone Mfg Co,
Ltd**
2-5-1, Akasaka
Minato-ku, Tokyo 107
Japan
Tel: +81 (3) 3583-8361
Fax: +81 (3) 3583-3328

**Telios Pharmaceuticals,
Inc**
4757 Nexus Centre Dr
San Diego, CA 92121
USA
Tel: +1 (619) 622-2600

**Teva Pharmaceuticals
(USA)**
650 Cathill Rd
PO Box 904
Sellersville, PA 18960
USA
Tel: +1 (215) 256-8400
Fax: +1 (215) 721-9669

Theraplix
Rhône-Poulenc Rorer
46-52, rue Albert
75640 Paris Cedex 13
France
Tel: +33 (1) 40 77 30 00
Fax: +33 (1) 40 77 322 20

Thomae GmbH, Dr Karl
Birkendorfer Str 65
88937 Biberach
Germany
Tel: +49 07351/54-0
Fax: +49 07351/54-4600

Tillots Pharma
Hauptstr 27
CH-4417 Ziefen
Switzerland

**Torii Pharmaceutical Co,
Ltd**
3-4-1, Nihonbashi
Hon-cho
Chuo-ku, Tokyo 103
Japan
Tel: +81 (3) 3231-6811
Fax: +81 (3) 5203-7333

Toyama Chemical Co, Ltd
3-2-5, Nishi-shinj u
Shinj u-ku, Tokyo 160
Japan
Tel: +81 (3) 5381-3889
Fax: +81 (3) 3348-6460

Toyo Jozo
Direct Inquiries to Asahi
Chemical

Toyo Koatsu Co, Ltd
Hiroshima
Japan

**Toyo Pharmachemicals
Co, Ltd**
Tokyo Bldg
2-7-3, Marunouchi
Chiyoda-ku, Tokyo 100
Japan
Tel: +81 (3) 3211-8621
Fax: +81 (3) 3211-8625

Trega Biosciences, Inc
3550 General Atomics Ct
San Diego, CA 92121
USA
Tel: +1 (619) 455-3814
Fax: +1 (619) 455-2544

Triple Crown America, Inc
13 N 7th St
Perkasie, PA 18944
USA
Tel: +1 (215) 453-2500
Fax: +1 (215) 453-2508

Troponwerke Dinklage
Address Unknown

US Bioscience Corp
One Tower Bridge
100 Front St
W Conshohocken, PA
19428
USA
Tel: +1 (610) 832-0570
Fax: +1 (610) 832-4500

US Ethicals, Inc
Address Unknown

US Vitamin
Address Unknown

UCB Pharma
Allee de la Recherche 60
Brussels
Belgium
Tel: +32 (2) 559 9999
Fax: +32 (2) 559 9900

UCB Pharma
21, rue de Neuilly
92003 Nanterre Cedex
France
Tel: +33 (1) 47 29 44 35
Fax: +33 (1) 47 25 47 20

Manufacturers and Suppliers Directory

UCB Pharma oy Finland
Maistraatinporti 2
FIN-0020 Helsinka
Finland

UCB Research, Inc
840 Memorial Dr
Cambridge, MA 02139
USA
Tel: + 1 (617) 547-8481

Ucyclyd Pharma, Inc
Direct Inquiries to Medicis
Pharmaceutical Corp

**Ueno Fine Chemicals
Industry, Ltd**
2-4-8, Koraibashi
Chuo-ku, Osaka 541
Japan
Tel: +81 (6) 6203-0761
Fax: +81 (6) 6222-2413

Ueno Kagaku Kogyo KK
3-3-2, Shodai Tajika
Hirakata-shi, Osaka 573
Japan
Tel: +81 (7) 20 56-2281

Ugine Kuhlmann
Direct Inquires to Rhône
Poulenc

Unicler
Address Unknown

Unilab Corp
401 Hackensack Ave
Hackensack, NJ
07601-6411
USA
Tel: +1 (201) 525-1000

Unilever International
Greyfriars
Lewins Mead
Bristol Avon BS1 2JJ
England
Tel: +44 (01272) 276276

**Unimed Pharmaceuticals,
Inc**
2150 East Lake Cook Rd
Ste 210
Buffalo Grove, IL
60089-1862
USA
Tel: +1 (847) 541-2525
Fax: +1 (847) 541-2569

Union Carbide Corp
Address Unknown
Danbury, CT
USA
Tel: +1 (203) 794-7024

United Catalysts Inc
PO Box 32370
Louisville, KY 40232
USA
Tel: +1 (502) 634-7200
Fax: +1 (502) 637-3132

Upjohn Ltd
Direct Inquiries to
Pharmacia & Upjohn

Uriach
Address Unknown

Usines de Melle
Direct Inquiries to Rhône
Poulenc

Valeas
via Vallisneri, 10
20133 Milano
Italy

Vanderbilt, RT Co Inc
30 Winfield
Enfield, CT 06082
USA
Tel: +1 (203) 853-1400

VEB Arzneimittelwerk
Address Unknown

VEB Farbenfabrik Wolfen
Address Unknown

Vismara
Address Unknown

Vistakon, Inc
4500 Salisbury Rd
Ste 300
Jackson, FL 32216
USA
Tel: +1 (904) 443-1000

**Wakamoto
Pharmaceutical Co, Ltd**
1-5-3, Nihonbahi
Muro-machi
Chuo-ku, Tokyo 103
Japan
Tel: +81 (3) 3279-0371
Fax: +81 (3) 3279-0393

Walker Labs
Address Unknown

Wallace & Tiernan, Inc
P O Box 178
Newark, NJ 07101-9976
USA
Tel: +1 (973) 759-8000
Fax: +1 (973) 751-6589

Wallace & Tiernan Ltd
Priory Works
Tonbridge
Kent TN11 0QL
England
Tel: +44 (01732) 771777
Fax: +44 (01732) 77190

Wallace Laboratories
10200 E Girard Ave
Denver, CO 80231-0550
USA
Tel: +1 (303) 745-4676

**Walter Reed Army
Institute of Research**
16th Street NW
Washington, DC 20307
USA

Walton Pharmaceuticals
Bowes House, Bowes Rd
Walton on Thames
Surrey
England
Tel: +44 (01923) 24103

Wander Pharma
Deutschherrnstr 15
90429 Nuernberg
Germany
Tel: +49 911 2730
Fax: +49 911 273653

Ward Blenkinsop
Address Unknown

Manufacturers and Suppliers Directory

Warner Lambert
201 Tabor Rd
Morris Plains, NJ 07950
USA
Tel: +1 (973) 385-2000

Wellcome Foundation Ltd, The
PO Box 129
Unicorn House
160 Euston Rd
London, NW1 2BP
England
Tel: +44 (020) 7387 4477

Wellcome plc
Unicorn House
160 Euston Rd
London, NW1 2BP
England
Tel: +44 (020) 7387 4477

Wesley-Jessen
333 East Howard Ave
Des Plaines, IL 60018
USA
Tel: +1 (847) 294-3000
Fax: +1 (847) 294-3434

Westwood-Squibb Pharmaceuticals, Inc
100 Forest Ave
Buffalo, NY 14213
USA
Tel: +1 (716) 887-3400

Whitefin Holding
Address Unknown

Whitehall
111, rue des Chateau des Rentiers
75013 Paris
France
Tel: +33 (1) 44 06 43 21
Fax: +33 (1) 44 06 43 69

Whitehall Laboratories Ltd
Huntercombe Lane South
Taplow
Maidenhead,
Berks SL6 0PH
England
Tel: +44 (01628) 669011

Whitehall Labs
111, rue des Chateau des Rentiers
75013 Paris
France
Tel: +33 (1) 44 06 43 21
Fax: +33 (1) 44 06 43 69

Whitehall-Robins
PO Box 8299
Philadelphia, PA 19101
USA
Tel: +1 (973) 660-6805

Wiernik AG
Address Unknown

Windsor Healthcare Ltd
Ellesfield Avenue
Bracknell
Berks RG12 8YS
England
Tel: +44 (01344) 484448

Winthrop
Direct Inquiries to Sanofi Winthrop

Winthrop-Stearns
Direct Inquiries to Sanofi Winthrop

Wisconsin Alumni Research Foundation
Address Unknown

Worthington Biochemical
Address Unknown

Wyeth Laboratories
Direct Inquires to Wyeth-Ayerst Laboratories

Wyeth-Ayerst Laboratories
PO Box 8299
Philadelphia, PA 19101
USA
Tel: +1 (610) 971-4980

Xenon Vision
Address Unknown

Xoma Corp
2910 Seventh St
Berkeley, CA 94710
USA
Tel: +1 (310) 829-7681

Xttrium Labs, Inc
415 West Pershing Rd
Chicago, IL 60609
USA
Tel: +1 (773) 268-5800
Fax: +1 (773) 924-6002

Yamanouchi Europe BV
PO Box 108
NL-2350 A C Leiderdrop
The Netherlands
Tel: +31 7154 55745
Fax: +31 7154 800

Yamanouchi Pharma
10, pl de la Coupole - BP 105
94223 Charenton Le Pont Cedex
France
Tel: +33 (1) 46 76 64 00
Fax: +33 (1) 46 76 64 99

Yamanouchi USA Inc
4747 Willow Rd
Pleasanton, CA 94588
USA
Tel: +1 (925) 924-2000

Yoshitomi
2-6-9, Hirano-machi
Chuo-ku, Osaka 541
Japan
Tel: +81 (6) 6201-2646
Fax: +81 (6) 6232-0910

Zambeletti
Address Unknown

Zambon France
46/48, avenue du General Leclerc
92100
Boulogne-Billancourt
France
Tel:+33 (1) 46 99 15 60

Zambon Group
Via Lillo del Duca, 10
Bresso
20091 Milano
Italy
Tel: +39 (02) 665241
Fax: +39 (02) 66501492

Zeeland Chemicals
215 N Centennial St
Zeeland, MI 49464
USA
Tel: +1 (616) 772-2193
Fax: +1 (616) 772-6554

Zeneca Pharmaceuticals
Alderley Park
Macclesfield
 Cheshire SK10 4TF
England
Tel: +44 (01625) 582828

Zeneca Pharmaceuticals
Kings Court
Water Lane
Wilmslow
Cheshire SK9 5AZ
England
Tel: +44 (01625) 712712